BE YOUR OWN DOCTOR

Dr. (Mrs.) KANTA GUPTA
M.A. LL.B. Ph.D.
Yogashiromani,
Jyotish Visharad

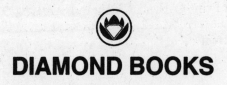

DIAMOND BOOKS

ISBN : 81-7182-031-X

© Publisher

Published by	:	**Diamond Pocket Books Pvt. Ltd.**
		X-30, Okhla Industrial Area, Phase-II
		New Delhi-110020
Phone	:	011-41611861
Fax	:	011-41611866
E-mail	:	sales@dpb.in
Website	:	www.dpb.in
Edition	:	2008
Printed by	:	Star Print-O-Bind, Okhla Ind. Area, N.D.-20

BE YOUR OWN DOCTOR
By: *Dr. (Mrs.) Kanta Gupta*

ABOUT THE AUTHOR

Materialism is order of the day and it seems as if the whole world is becoming sickeningly materialistic. Still there is a ray of hope in the form of those handful of people who truly believe that Eternal bliss or Nirvana or Moksha can never be attained so long as the mind and the body crave for all that is material. Such people do full justice to their family, profession and other social obligations and still find time for serving humanity, practising meditation & introspection & following their literary pursuits.

Such one person, who is most apt to fit in the above framework, who is principled, dedicated, educated, endowed with more virtues than most people ever dream of is: 'Dr. Mrs. Kanta Gupta' — She is 'PARAM YOGINI' in the real sense. Like the lotus, which radiates its beauty although it might be surrounded by filth, she shines amongst the millions, who might be billionaires but are paupers as far as virtues, priorities, principles and dedication to the welfare of humanity goes.

Her life partner Shri Rajiv Lochan, son of a great philanthropist, due to saintly temperament and behaviour is called 'Mahatmaji' by us. Both of them have devoted many years of their lives to propogate the 'holy science of Yoga', They have not only allowed free use of office space in their house for different activities of Maharshi Dayanand Yogashram Society, of which Dr. Kanta is the 'Secretary General, — but also play host to all those Yoga- Devotees, who come there. The Zeal in helping in the organisation of the Ist World Yoga Conference and the hospitality accorded by the couple was truly Indian culture and hospitality at its best and those memories are cherished by all the delegates who attended the conference.

Dr. Kanta worked consistently to Write an illustrated Encyclopedia on Yoga — entitled 'Yoga Nidhi', which contains the history of Yoga right from beginning of Civilisation till date. This compilation is undoubtedly the result of her persistent devotion and untiring efforts.

She is a renowned scholar of ancient Indian culture and her academic contribution specially in the field of socio- economic-legal aspects of status of women reflect her multi-faceted learning and analytical research acumen. Her extensive visits to several countries all over the world - U.S.A. Mauritius, Canada, Austria, Italy, France, Switzerland, U.K., Australia, Hongkong, Singapore, Bangkok etc. has opened a new horizon in her academic vision and pursuits

She has been activety associated with the publication of 'Yoga Mandir' a monthly magazine and has been regularly contributing articles about the medicinal value of herbs, Vegetables, fruits etc. These articles became very popular and acclaimed to be of great utility. On persistent demand from the public, she has laboured hard to compile them in a book form entitled 'Be your own doctor'.

In this book "Be your own doctor" she has given a very vivid and graphic description of various herbs, vegetables, trees, condiments etc. emphasizing their utility, efficacy and medicinal properties. Written in simple, lucid and easy flowing style this book will prove extremely beneficial for one and all.

With these words. I pray to All Mighty God to shower his blessings on Dr. Kanta and give her strength and great success in the attainment of noble objects, she is working for.

ACHARYA BHAGWAN DEV
EX M.P
CHANCELLOR
Gurukul University, Brindavan — 281121

FOREWORD

"धर्मार्थकाममोक्षाणामारोग्यं मूलमुत्तमम्"—i.e. for complete fulfilment of all the four-fold ends of human life — a healthy body is the most essential.

Modern living has started taking its heavy toll. Constant stress, insatiable desires and ambitions, sophisticated artificial life-style, mad race to be on the top, extreme atmospheric pollution has resulted in producing more and more "mental" and "physical " ailments. Every second person is suffering from one problem or other — starting from simple indigestion, headaches to heart trouble, cancer, Aids etc. etc. The list is endless. Moreover, the disease that strikes the person gets aggravated till one really takes out spare time to go to a doctor or hospital. Apart from non-availability of treatment at the earliest — the medicines are very costly and sometimes beyond the reach of poor people (who constitute the majority of our population). Efficacy of most of the medicines is still questionable vis-a-vis the side effects. As a matter of fact, prolonged use of several medicines promotes the growth of many other complications.

What then...? What is the cure...? To nip the disease in the bud. "GO BACK TO NATURE & BE YOUR OWN DOCTOR". In this book I have undertaken to highlight the composition, therapeutic properties and different uses of some very commonly available trees, fruits, vegetables, plants and condiments. The most important aspect of it is that they are readily available to everyone irrespective of the place or status. Regular use in proper proportion will help in preventing the disease and keeping fit and healthy.This book will become a permanent companion. The more it is read and used, the more helpful it will prove.

I must acknowledge gratitude to Acharya Bhagwan Dev Ex M.P, Chancellor , Gurukul University, Brindavan U.P for providing guidance and taking keen interest in my work.

I am particularly indebted to my husband Sh. Rajiv Lochan, who has always been a source of inspiration for pursuing my research and has given me great help in compiling this book.

I am sincerely thankful to Bhai Narendraji — Director Diamond Pocket Books, Darya Ganj, Delhi, for publishing this book — thus making it possible to reach the readers all over the world.

The ultimate purpose of this book is to make the entire humanity — embodiment of "सत्यं शिवं सुन्दरम्" i.e. all that is Truthful, all that is Benevolent and all that is Beautiful".

2, Park Avenue, Maharani Bagh,   DR. (Mrs.) KANTA GUPTA
New Delhi-110 065
INDIA

CONTENTS

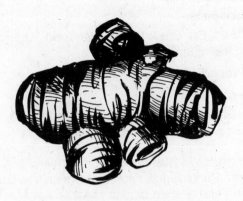

ADARAK (Ginger)

1. Adarak is known in different languages as—

1.	Sanskrit	—	*Ardraka, Katubhadra, Sringavera*
2.	Hindi	—	*Adarak, Adarakh*
3.	Latin	—	*Zingiber officinate*
4.	Bengali	—	*Ada*
5.	Marathi	—	*Ala*
6.	Kannada	—	*Alla*
7.	Telegu	—	*Allam*
8.	Gujrati	—	*Adun*
9.	Tamil	—	*Inji*
10.	Sindhi	—	*Adarak*
11.	English	—	*Ginger root*

2. Description—

Ginger plant is 1.2 ft. in height with long leaves and mauve-coloured flower. The underground part known as 'Rhizome' is the edible part and is called 'Ginger-root'. It is grown in barren or sandy soil and is wheatish in colour. Fresh form is called 'Ginger' and the dried form 'Sonth' (dried ginger-root)

It is pungent and a bit bitter in taste. It acts as digestive, carminative, stomachic, anti-pyreutic, generates heat, expels flatus and cough, purifies blood and is invigorating.

It is given in atonic dyspepsia, chronic bronchical cough and palpitation of heart. It is corrective to nauseous medicines and analgesic. It checks griping due to purgative and is needed as flavouring adjuvant.

3. Its Composition is –

Volatile Oil-2% Fat, Crude Liquid; Oleo-resin gingerol or gingerin; Mucilage; Resin; Starch 20%; Ash 4%

4. Curative Properties –

Asthma, Cough

(i) 1 tsp. mixture of juice of ginger. lahsun and honey (in equal quantity) taken 2-3 times a day-relieves bronchial Congestion, cures Cough & gives relief.

(ii) Sucking 1 Goli (Heat Powdered Sonth and Black pepper 10 Gms. each in 100 gm. Gur-till it gets thick. Make gram size Goli) 4-6 times a day cures coughing and relieves pain in chest and stomach due to constant cough.

(iii) Heated ginger juice with honey (1 tsp each) 3 times a day for few days cures cold & cough and gives relief in Asthma.

(iv) 10 gms of ginger pieces boiled in water taken with sugar and milk like tea 2-3 times a day cures cold & cough.

Digestive & Stomach Problems

(i) 2 tsp of juice (of ginger, fresh lemon and honey in equal quantity) taken early in the morning helps in digestion, increases appetite and improves blood circulation.

(ii) Chatni of Ginger, fresh coriander leaves with Sendha Namak & Black Pepper taken half an hour before meals cures indigestion.

(iii) 6 gms ginger piece with Sendha Namak taken before meals for 10 days relieves flatulence.

(iv) Churna of Sonth (dried ginger), Heeng and Sendha Namak taken after meals acts as a digestive.

(v) Small pieces of fresh ginger fried in pure ghee with little salt twice a day cures indigestion. Taking 1 tsp churna (finely powdered Sonth, Ajwayan and Black Pepper (10 gms. each), Kala Namak, choti Illayachi, Sugar (5 gms.each) to be strained and kept as Churna) after meals cures all stomach and digestive problems.

(vi) Prepare decoction by boiling pieces of ginger, Dhania seeds, little Jeera, 8-10 Kishmish in 1.5 kg. water till it is reduced to 250 gm. Strain it and mix it with Mishri, Taking this cures bile and helps in digestion.

(vii) Drinking milk with pieces of ginger boiled in it eliminates wind & cures intestinal problems.

(viii) 1.5 tsp. ginger juice acts as an adjuvant to laxatives (castor-oil etc.) and checks gripping.

Diarrhoea:

$\frac{1}{2}$ tsp. juice of ginger mixed with half cup of boiled water-taken 3-4 times a day cures loose motions.

Hiccough:

Chewing and sucking the juice of small pieces of ginger, or taking $\frac{1}{2}$ tsp. powdered dried sonth boiled in milk stops hiccough.

Hoarseness of throat

(i) Taking $\frac{1}{2}$ tsp. ginger juice with honey 3-4 times a day or chewing and sucking little ginger piece 3-4 times a day cures hoarseness of throat.

(ii) Make a hole in ginger and fill it with little heeng, wrap this in cloth and heat it. After grinding it, make small balls like chana and take this tablet 4-5 times a day. It cures hoarseness of throat.

Influenza

(i) Taking decoction (made of 3 gms of sonth, 7 Tulsi leaves, 7 Black pepper seeds boiled in 250 gms. water with sugar to taste) cures cold, cough, headache and gives relief in Influenza.

(ii) $\frac{1}{2}$ tsp. of powdered Sonth with little sendha Namak 3-4 times a day with hot water relieves sputum.

Pain in Ribs

Taking sonth decoction by boiling 20 gms. of Sonth in $\frac{1}{2}$ kg. water to be taken in 4 doses cures pain in ribs.

Back-ache, Menstural Disorder

(i) Taking 1 dose of Churna (1 gm. powdered Sonth, 1.5 gm. Meetha Soda mixed with 2 gm. salt heated on Tawa to be taken in 4 doses) with hot milk or water before going to bed cures backache.

(ii) Taking decoction of powdered Sonth with old Ghee cures back- ache & regulates menstural disorders.

Headache

Fomentation with paste of powdered Sonth made with warm water on the forehead cures headache.

Ear-ache—1 drop of Ginger oil (ginger juice boiled in mustard oil) put in ear relieves ear-ache.

Arthritis

Taking 10 gms of Sonth boiled in 100 gms water with Shakkar or Gur for some time cures Arthrites.

Paralysis

(i) Fry paste of ground Urad Dal. mix Sonth and Gur and make Laddu. Eating one Laddu daily helps in curing paralysis.

(ii) Boil Urad Dal with little sonth in water for some time. Drinking this water cures paralysis.

Numbness of Limbs

(i) Applying paste of Sonth and Lahsun (with water) on the affected limb cures numbness.

(ii) Chewing little Sonth with 2 Shellots of Lahsun early in the morning for 10-15 days improves circulation of blood and cures numbness.

Obesity

Taking 2 gms. of Churna (Sonth, Pippali, Black Pepper 100 gms. each; Dhania seeds, Kala Jeera 10 gms. each; Kala Namak, Sendha Namak, Pahari Namak 5 gms. each; to be powdered and kept as Churna) twice a day after meals cures obesity.

(*Note* — To Keep ginger fresh, cover the Rhizome with sand or mud and sprinkle water everyday on it.)

Precautions

Ginger stimulates and generates heat and therefore should be taken very carefully in summer and autumn season.

Note — ill effects of ginger are eliminated by taking honey or almond oil.

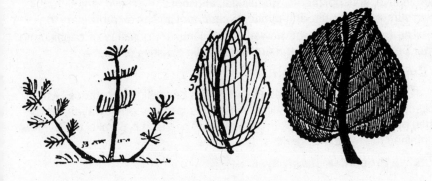

AJAWAYAN
(Beshops Weed Seed)

1. Ajawayan is known in different languages as : —

1.	Sanskrit	—	*Yavani, Yavanika, Ugra-gandha, Dipyaka, Dipya*
2.	Hindi	—	*Ajawayan*
3.	Latin	—	*Ptychotis Ajawayan*
4.	Bengali	—	*Yamani, Yoyama*
5.	Marathi	—	*Ova*
6.	Kannada	—	*Ondie*
7.	Telegu	—	*Vamu*
8.	Gujarati	—	*Yavana, Jawaina*
9.	Tamil	—	*Amana*
10.	Sindhi	—	*Ajwayana*
11.	English	—	*Beshops Weed Seed.*

2. Description : —

The height of Ajawayan plant is 3-4 ft. It is cultivated in black soil particularly along the riverbanks throughout India. It has small leaves and white inflorescence. From these flowers we get thousands of seeds – known as Ajawayan.

13

Ajawayan is pungent and bitter in taste. It is a great stimulant, carminative, antisposmodic, germicidal, antiseptic, digestive, anti-flatulent, heart stimulant, diuretic, anti-pyritic, expectorant and an extraordinary tonic.

The fruit combines the powerful and stimulant qualities of capsicum, bitter property of Chiretta and anti-spasmodic qualities of Heeng.

3. Composition of Ajawayan : –

It contains an aromatic volatile oil and a crystalline substance, which collects on the surface of distilled water. This is flower of Ajawayan, which when ripened assumes the form of Ajawayan seeds. It is parallel to Thymol contained in Thymus Vulgaris.

Curative Properties of Ajawayan : –

Flatulence, Indigestion, Low Appetite : –

As an antispasmodic, regular use of Ajawayan is recommended.

(i) Take $\frac{1}{2}$ tsp. Aqua Ptychotis (Sat) of Ajawayan mixed with water morning and evening.

(ii) Take 1 tsp. of mixture (made of 4 tsp. Aqua Ptychotis with 4 tsp. Lemon juice and 5 drops of Ilayachi Ark) thrice a day.

(iii) Take 1 tsp. of Churn (prepared with ground Ajawayan and small Harr-equal quantity, little Heeng and Salt to taste) with hot water after meals.

(iv) Swallow 3 gms. of ground Ajawayan with $\frac{3}{4}$ gm. of Kaala Namak twice a day.

(v) Take $\frac{1}{2}$ tsp. of Churna (made of Ajawayan, Black Pepper, Saunth taken in equal quantity) morning and evening with water.

(vi) Take Ajawayan seeds soaked in lime juice after meals. This helps in digestion.

Strangury : –

Taking 2 gms. of Ajawayan with 3 gms. of Mishri twice or thrice a day relieves strangury.

Polyuria : –

(i) Taking 1 tsp. Ajawayan with Til in equal quantity twice a day eliminates polyuria.

(ii) 1 tsp. powder (of Ajawayan and Gur-equal quantity) taken 4 times a day relieves polyuria and cures pain in Kidneys.

Bronchitis and Asthma: –

(i) Taking 1 tsp. Ajawayan with hot water morning and evening lessens sputum.

(ii) Fomentation of chest with hot seeds tied as poultice lessens sputum.

Cold and Cough :—

(i) Rubbing the palm with 6 gms. of Ajawayan tied in a potli and smelling it repeatedly cures cold.

(ii) Drinking hot water after chewing little Ajawayan cures cough.

(iii) Taking $\frac{1}{2}$ tsp. Aqua Ptychotis with little salt relieves constant cough.

(iv) Chewing betel leaf with Ajawayan at night before sleeping controls and cures dry coughing.

Influenza :—

(i) Drinking boiled water with 3 gms. Ajawayan and 3 gms. Dalcheeni for 3 to 4 days-thrice a day cures influenza.

(ii) Drinking decoction (made with 2-3 gms. Ajawayan boiled in 3 cups of water till a cup remains) — 4 times a day for 2-3 days cures influenza.

Diarrhoea and stomach-ache :—

(i) Take Ajawayan and salt in the ratio of 2;1 with hot water. It cures stomach-ache, improves digestion and controls diarrhoea.

(ii) Take 1 tsp. of Churna of Ajawayan, Sendha Namak, black pepper, Illayachi and roasted small Harr (1 gm. each) after meals.

(iii) Take 1 gm. powder (made with 15 gms. Ajawayan, 5 gms. Kaala Namak and $\frac{1}{2}$ gm. Heeng) with hot water twice a day.

(iv) Take little Ajawayan with Camphor with water twice a day.

Tooth-ache :—

(i) Give smoke to the aching tooth by burning Ajawayan on fire and after 2 hours (of smoke) do gargles with lukewarm water (prepared by boiling 1 tsp. gound Ajawayan with little salt) two to three times a day. It cures tooth-ache.

Ear-ache :—

Putting one or two drops of Ajawayan oil relieves ear ache.

Heart-ache :—

Taking 1 tsp. Ajawayan with hot water stimulates the heart and relieves heart-ache.

Throat-ache :—

Doing gargles with lukewarm Ajawayan water (made by boiling 1 tsp. ground Ajawayan with little salt in water) twice or thrice cures coarseness and pain in throat.

Rheumatic pains, Arthritis :—

(i) Poultice of crushed Ajawayana applied to painful rheumatic joints relieves pain.

(ii) Massage of affected portion with Ajawayan oil relieves pain.

Foul Ulcers, Ringworm, Itchings : —

(i) Taking Ajawayan flower (in little quantity) acts as an antiseptic killing germs.

(ii) Cleaning the affected part with Ajawayan water kills the germs.

(iii) Applying paste of Ajawayan ground with hot water helps in curing ring-worm, itching and removes offensive smell from foul ulcers.

Stomach worms : —

(i) Taking 3 to 7 drops of Ajawayan oil for few days destroys worms in stomach.

(ii) Taking Ajawayan Churna with Chacha is also useful.

(iii) Boil 25 gms. ground Ajawayan soaked over night in 500 gm. water till 125 gm. water remains.

Taking this decoction (as 1 dose) twice a day for 2-3 days- destroys worms.

The same is to be divided and given in 2 doses for children.

Bile

Taking 2 gms. of Ajawayan with 3 gm. of Gur — in winter season — cures bile.

Menstrual disorders and post-natal care : —

(i) 6 gms. Churna of Ajawayana with hot milk regulates the menstrual flow of blood.

(ii) Eating Laddus of Ajawayan (- Soak-washed, dried ground desi Ajawayan in Desi Ghee for 1-2 weeks. Fry 1 kg Suji in pure ghee and mix 250 gm. Ajawayan and Khand to taste) after delivery.

or

Taking ground Ajawayan with Gur after delivery for few days relieves back-ache, cleans the uterus, stimulates digestion, increases appetite and gives strength.

Leucorrhoea : —

Taking paste of Ajawayan (25 gms. soaked in 125 gms. of water in earthen pot overnight and ground with water) in the morning for some time controls leucorrhoea.

Female Infertility : —

(i) Taking paste of Ajawayan (25 gms. of Ajawayan and 25 gms. Mishri soaked in 125 gms. water in earthen pot overnight-ground like Thandai paste) with water for 8-10 days in the morning (starting from Ist day of menses) and (ii) having mung ki Dal (without Salt and Chappatis in meals helps in curing infertility.

Pimples :‒

Applying paste of 30 gms. or ground Ajawayan mixed with 25 gms. curd on face at night and washing the face in the morning with hot water-cures pimples and brings glow to the face. /

Urticaria :‒

Taking 1 gm. ground Ajawayan with 3 gms. of Gur-relieves Urticaria.

Stones :‒

Taking 3-4 gms. of Ajawayan daily for sometime with water help in breaking the stones and its expulsion from kidney or urinary bladder.

Wind :‒

Taking 1 tsp. ground Ajawayan with $\frac{1}{4}$ tsp. Kaala Namak in skimmed curd -relieves wind.

Whooping cough :‒

Taking 1 gm. paste (made by mixing ground 20 gms. Ajawayan 5 gms. Kaala Namak in 60-70 gms. honey) 3 or 4 times regularly helps in curing whooping cough.

As Deodorant :‒

Ajawayan is very effective in killing the germs and insects and purifies the air.

Keeping a potlie of Ajawayan in cubboard infested with cock- roaches etc. helps in killing them.

Apart from its inherent curative properties Ajawayan is cheap and easily available in every kitchen. Its regular use is very beneficial and does not result in any mental or physical side-affects.

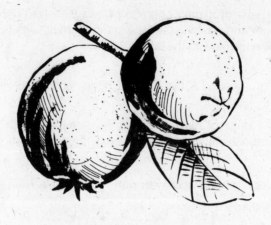

AMRUDA (Guava)

1. Amruda is known in different languages as: –

1.	Sanskrit	–	*Amruda*
2.	Hindi	–	*Amruda*
3.	Latin	–	*Psidium Guayava*
4.	Bengali	–	*Goachi*
5.	Marathi	–	*Jamba*
6.	Kannada	–	*Sive*
7.	Telegu	–	*Jama, Goya*
8.	Gujrati	–	*Jamarukha, Peru*
9.	Tamil	–	*Koyya, Segappugoyya*
10.	Sindhi	–	*Jetuna*
11.	English	–	*Guava*

2. Description: –

Guava is one of the famous and well known fruits grown all over India, especially in U.P. Its tree is of medium height. It bears fruits twice in a year- in summers and winter but the fruit in winter is superior in quality and taste. Different varieties of guava are available but the best is that which is grown around Allahabad. It has few seeds and is very delicious and tasty.

The pulp of guava is very useful for human system. It is digestive, carminative, giver of vigour and strength to heart, lungs and the body. It is an effective aphrodis, improves blood-circulation, heals and dries wound and is an antiseptic.

3. Its Chemical Composition is : –

Protein	1.5%
Fat	0.2%
Minerals	0.8%
Carbohydrates	14.5%
Calcium	1.01%
Phosphorous	0.44%
Iron	1.0 mg. per gram.
Vitamin B	0.2
Vitamin c	2.99 mg.

It has 20 units of Vitamin 'A', 10 units of Vitamin B, fluid Isopelletierine, alkaline and watery contents. Thus a medium sized Guava is a source of about 70-80 calories.

4. Curative Properties of Guava

1. General Tonic: –

(i) Taking 200 gm. ripe guava with kaala Namak, black-pepper and little lemon juice-twice a day regularly-gives strength and vigour to mental and physical muscles.

(ii) Taking ripe guava with fig (Anjeer) and Tulsi leaves after meals checks physical nervousness.

(iii) Taking guava pulp and banana pulp with honey in breakfast eliminates the look of lanky body by making it grow strong and sturdy.

(iv) Taking peeled and cut cheekus and guava with honey twice a day gives a lot of strength to the body.

Blood-impurities : –

Taking 200 gm. well ripe Guava with mid day meals daily-purifies blood and also improves haemoglobin.

Nausea: –

Taking juice of Guava leaves or half raw & half ripe Guava (with Sendha Namak & lime-juice) cures nausea.

Headache : –

(i) Applying paste of ground green leaves of Guava with little sandal wood on the forehead for half an hour eliminates headache.

(ii) Eating a fresh ripe guava after taking out its seeds is also useful.

Migraine : –

Applying ground pulp of unripe Guava on the affected part early in the morning - for 2 days - eliminates Migraine pain.

High Blood-Pressure : —

Taking the oozed out water of the chaat made of Guavas with little Sendha Namak, black pepper, lemon-juice on it-twice or thrice a week checks high blood-pressure.

Throat Problems : —

(i) Gargling with Guava leaves water & salt - (fresh guava leaves to be boiled in 400 gm. water till it is reduced to 125 gm.: strain it) twice or thrice cures sore-ness of throat.

(ii) Taking ripe Guava pulp with little honey & black pepper-clears the throat infection.

Cough : —

Taking baked Guava (after removing seeds) with honey twice a day controls phlegm.

Digestive and stomach problems : —

(i) Taking pulp of roasted Guava (after taking out seeds) with orange juice-two or three times a day-cures indigestion.

(ii) Taking Guava with Sendha Namak after meals-eliminates gas & increases appetite.

(iii) Taking ground paste of 8-10 Guava fresh leaves with water cures stomach-ache.

Constipation : —

(i) Taking Guava in breakfast or before meals activates digestion and cures constipation.

(ii) Taking Guava pulp, papaya pulp with little black pepper, Sendha Namak and lemon juice sprinkled on it-after meals activates normal movement of bowels.

(iii) Taking ripe Guava after meals is also very useful.

Loose Motions : —

(i) Taking boiled water of Guava leaves-2 or 3 times a day controls loose motions.

(ii) Taking ripe guava after lunch with sprinkling of sendha Namak, black-pepper and lemon juice helps in proper digestion.

(iii) Guava Chutney with meals is useful.

Arthritis : —

(i) Taking juice of soft red leaves of Guava plant-with water twice a day relieves stiffness of joints.

(ii) Applying of paste of Guava leaves on the affected parts eliminates swelling.

Itching : –

Regularly taking 250 gms. ripe Guava in the afternoon for about 1 month purifies blood, cleans the stomach and intestines and thus cures itching due to bowls, pustules etc.

Wounds : –

Applying paste of Guava leaves-on wounds helps in curing the wound.

Urinary troubles : –

Taking decoction of leaves of 10 gm. Guava and 50 gm. Grapes (Heat theses leaves with 600 gm. water till it is half-strain it) before sleep eliminates and cures all urinary troubles.

Piles : –

Eating Guavas regularly helps in curing piles.

Worms : –

(i) Taking the pulp of roasted Guava (after removing seeds) with 3-4 drops of garlic juice for one or two days-on empty stomach helps in expelling the dead worms.

(ii) Taking pulp of roasted Guava & a Tomato (after removing seeds) with little Sendha Namak and few drops of lemon juice empty stomach in the morning-helps in expulsion of dead worms.

Tooth-ache : –

Chewing fresh Guava leaves or doing gargles with Guava leaves water (in which guava leaves are boiled) eliminates swelling of gums and cures tooth-ache.

Other Uses : –

(i) Apart from the curative properties its wood is very hard and used for making Harmonium etc. on which carving can also be done.

(ii) The bark and dry leaves are used for making dyes for clothes.

Guava, because of its nutritive value, is also used as food-item. Guava sharbat, Guava Jam, Guava Juice are commonly used as appetiser and tasty drink especially in summers.

Rich in Calories Guava has many qualities of apple and is rightly called 'POORMAN'S APPLE'.

Precautions : –

(i) Guava should not be taken empty stomach because it give rise to phlegm in the body.

(ii) Don't drink water after eating Guava for it may lead to cholera.

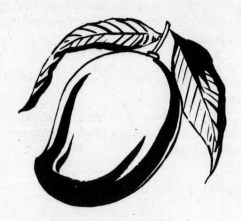

AAM (Mango)

1. Mango is known in different languages as :—

1.	Sanskrit	—	*Amra, Chuta, Rasala, Sahakara, Kamanga*
2.	Hindi	—	*Aam*
3.	Latin	—	*Mangifera Indica*
4.	Bengali	—	*Aam, Amra*
5.	Marathi	—	*Anwa, Amba*
6.	Kannada	—	*Mavinphala*
7.	Telegu	—	*Mamidi,*
8.	Gujrati	—	*Ambo*
9.	Tamil	—	*Mangai*
10.	Sindhi	—	*Amb*
11.	English	—	*Mango*

2. Description :—

Mango is undisputed and uncrowned king of all the fruits. It is found all over India. Its tree is about 40-50 ft. high with black skin and dark-brown rind or bark over it. It starts giving fruit only after 5 or 6 years. Various varieties of Mango are available as — Kalami, Dussahri (U.P), Langda (Benaras), Desi Aam, Alphanso (Bombay), Safeda (Lucknow U.P), Chausa (U.P) and many many others.

Its taste is sweet and little sour, and is very, nourishing. Its name 'Amritphala' in ancient treatises-bespeaks of its great nutritive value. Its qualities vary with growth. Raw mango is sour and stringent and produces wind and bile. The pealed raw mangoes cut in pieces are dried in sun & that becomes Amchoor. Amchoor is sour and stringent in taste & is carminative, antiphlegm.atic and checks wind problems. Ripe Mango is extremely tasty and nutritive fruit. A normal sized mango is more nourishing for the human body than butter or almonds. It strengthens and invigorates all the nerves, tissues, muscles in the brain, heart and other parts of the body. It is 'Tridoshanashak' anti-bileous, anti-phlegm.atic and antiacidic. It is carminative, digestive, general tonic, aphrodisiac, vermifuge, blood-purifier. It cleans the body of the filth within and is an ideal antidote for all toxic effects inside the body.

Medicinally Desi sweet Aam is the best. Sucking the juice and not eating cut-pieces is better for health. Mango-milk is an ideal combination because milk provides protein, which is lacking in mango and makes it "full meal". Not only does it keep the body in good and healthy shape, but also it provides sufficient resistance to fight any germs and afflictions.

Mango is not only liked and relished as fruit but many tasty, delicious preparations are made from raw and ripe mangoes like salads, chutney, murabba, pickles, Aamras, Halwa, Burfi, Kulfi, Aam papad, Shreekhanda etc. Every part of the mango tree-root, stemis, bark, the blossom, fruits have curative and medicinal properties. Apart from these it has many other uses: —

(i) Aam leaves are tied and decorated as 'Vandanvar' on all religious and auspicious occasions.

(ii) Aam twig is kept in utensil full of water on auspicious ceremonies.

(iii) Aam's wood is considered very pure for sacrifices.

(iv) Blossoms of Mango (Manjari) is offered to Gods.

(v) Its wood is used for making doors, stools, & other furniture.

(vi) Dried leaves are used as fuel.

(vii) Manure prepared with the help of rotten leaves is used in fields.

Thus Mango is the real "King of Fruits".

Antidote :—

Antidote against eating too many mangoes is

(i) Have few Jamuns over it.

(ii) Take cuminseeds water over it.

(iii) Sonth powder with water over it.

(iv) Ground roasted Jeera with Rock Salt over it.

Note :—

(i) Mango should not be taken empty stomach.

(ii) Too much intake of mangoes leads to indigestion, constipation, gaseous troubles, blood impurities & eye-troubles.

(iii) Water should never be taken after eating mangoes.

3. Chemical properties of Mango : –

Mango is rich in vitamin A & C and also has a little of vitamin B. For 100 gms. of pulp – it has 4500 I.U. Vitamin A.

Apart from this-Ripe Mango has : –

86. 1% water, 11. 8% Carbohydrates, 6% protein, 3% mineral salts 1% Fat. 0. 02% Phosphorous, 0. 01% calcium, 5mg iron per 100 gms. It also has fructose, citric acid, Tartaric Acid & Folic Acid. A normal sized mango gives 50 calories.

4. Curative properties of Mango : –

General Tonic : –

(i) Taking Mango pulp mixed in milk or drinking milk after eating mango imparts energy, strength and vigour to the body.

(ii) Taking juice of mango regularly in the evening eliminates physical weakness and improves nervous system.

(iii) Taking Mango or mango murabba after meals-helps in gaining weight and acts as a general tonic.

Mental weakness : –

Taking 1 cup Mango juice with 1 cup milk, 1 tsp. ginger juice, sugar to taste-daily eliminates mental weakness and strengthens the heart.

Hair problems : –

Massaging the hair with Mango oil (by cooking Kernel of a Mango stone in billing mustard oil. Cool it, strain & store) one or two hours before washing stops untimely greying of hair.

Headache : –

Applying the ground Kernel of Mango and a small Harar in milk (preferably of a goat) on the forehead gives immediate relief.

Anaemia : –

Taking mango and milk regularly eliminates anaemia.

Indigestion and stomach problems : –

(i) Sucking the juice of mango followed by milk regularly eliminates constipation and indigestion.

(ii) Taking 70 gms. of Mango juice and 2 gms. ground sonth in the morning-improves appetite and cures indigestion.

(iii) Licking ground powder of Mango Kernel with honey or boora in the same proportion gives instant relief in acidity.

(iv) Chewing few pieces or sucking the juice of raw mango eliminates indigestion due to fish-eating.

Loss of Appetite :–

(i) Taking the juice of Desi Aam with little rock salt and sugarcandy-twice a day helps in restoring lost appetite.

(ii) Taking Mango Murabba after meals is also very useful.

Diarrohea :–

(i) Taking $\frac{1}{2}$ cup sweet mango juice with 25 gms. curd and 1 tsp. ginger juice 2 or 3 times a day- controls loose motions.

(ii) Taking decoction of the bark of Mango (Boil 20 gms. powder of Mango bark in 1 kg water till 250 gms. is left) with 1 gm. Kaala Namak twice or thrice a day is also useful.

(iii) Taking 10 to 15 gms. ground powder of mango stone 2 or 3 times a day cures loose motions.

(iv) Applying the paste of mangostone on the navel also is helpful.

Dysentry :–

(i) Taking 20 gms. juice of fresh leaves of Mango with goat's milk (preferably) and honey 3 times a day helps in checking dysentery.

(ii) Taking the paste of rind of mango tree with honey twice a day checks dysentery.

(iii) Taking 2 gms. ground powder of stones of mango and Jamun (in equal proportion) with equal amount of Khandsari sugar-thrice a day with water-is also very useful.

(iv) Taking powder of stone of Mango with whey is also recommended.

(v) Taking $\frac{1}{2}$ tsp. ground powder of the leaves of Mango (dried in shade) with water 2 or 3 times a day is also useful.

Vomitting :–

Taking decoction of the seed of Mango (20 gm. crushed Guthli to be boiled in 1 kg water till 250 gms. water is left) with Desi Shakkar and honey-two times a day-controls vomiting.

Nausea during pregnancy :–

Sucking desi sweet mango gives instant relief.

Excessive Thirst :–

(i) Taking $\frac{1}{2}$ tsp. ground Kernel of the Mango stone with sugarcandy mixed in water 3 or 4 times a day controls excessive thirst.

(ii) Taking 10 gms. ground paste of fresh leaves of mango with honey-3 or 4 times a day-checks this.

Eye-problems : –

(i) Sucking the juice of sweet Desi Aaam-helps in curing Night-blindness.

(ii) Tying the poultice of mango pulp (by grinding raw mango's pulp and heating it a little) over the aching eye-eliminates pain, redness and irritation in the eye.

Tooth Problems : –

(i) Applying the powder of seed of mango-as tooth paste on teeth strengthens the gums and helps in curing all dental problems-foul smell, pyorrhoea etc.

(iii) Applying the ashes of burnt dry leaves of mango with little mustard oil and salt-as tooth paste-makes the gums and teeth strong and shining.

Hoarse Throat : –

Sipping decoction of the leaves of Mango mixed with honey-gives instant relief & clears the voice.

Dry Cough : –

Sucking the juice of a mango roasted on hot sand-clears all the bronchial congestions and gives relief.

Beauty-aid : –

Taking mango regularly makes the complexion fair and skin soft and shining.

Ezema : –

Applying the paste of mango mixed with little rock salt and oil on the affected parts-gives quick relief.

Spleen problems : –

Taking 50-60 gms. of Mango juice and 10-15 gms. honey regularly in the morning eliminates swelling and enlargement of spleen.

Stones : –

Taking 8 gms. finely ground powder of leaves of mango (fresh leaves dried in shade) with water (kept in a glass overnight) daily-helps in breaking the stones and throwing them out.

Liver troubles : –

Taking one drop of raw mango (dropped from its 'Chenp' the point with which it remains joined with the tree) in a Batasha-helps in curing liver problems.

(ii) Having tea of mango leaves (in place of tea-leaves) is also useful.

Insomnia :—

Taking sweet Desi Aam followed by lukewarm milk at night-helps in inducing sleep.

Diabetes :—

Taking juice of Mango and Jamun (in equal proportion) is good in controlling diabetes.

Piles :—

(i) Taking the juice of the inner side of rind of mango-stem daily is useful.

(ii) Taking ground powder of stone of mango 2 or 3 times a day is good.

(iii) Taking 20 gms. ground powder of Kernel of mango stone with whey for few days-is advisable.

Night-discharge :—

Applying the juice of Mango mixed with Alum powder and Nausador below navel before going to bed helps in eliminating this problem.

Leucorrohea :—

Taking decoction of inside of the bark of Mango tree (1 kg inside portion of the bark to be boiled in 5 kg water till $1\frac{1}{2}$ kg is left) mixed with sugarcandy or sugar to taste regularly 2 or 3 times a day, eliminates problem of discharge.

Gout :—

Massaging the affected part with powder of the Kernel of Mango stone mixed in mustard oil-eliminates pain.

Eruptions due to heat :—

Rubbing raw mango over these eruptions gives instant relief.

Worms :—

(i) Taking powder of Kernel of Mango-with warm warter-kills worms.

(ii) Taking powder of the mango stone mixing it with whey is also useful.

(iii) Taking decoction of Rind of Mangoes (boiled in water) after dinner kills and clears the worms in the stomach.

Asthma :—

Taking 5 gms. of powdered Kernel of Mango with water 2-3 times a day is useful in Asthma.

Eating Soil :—

(i) Taking powdered Kernel of Mango stone with fresh water cures the habit of eating soil in kids.

(ii) Taking roasted Kernel of Mango stone like supare-is also useful.

Poisonous Insect Bite : —

(i) Rubbing the mangostones's semi liquid paste (stone rubbed on wet surface to obtain paste) on the part bitten by scorpion, honeybee, wasp, mad dog, monkey etc. will eliminate the burning sensation and pain.

(ii) Applying dry Amchoor powder mixed in water on the affected part cures the spider burn.

Rickety : —

(i) Giving dried Amchoor powder soaked in pure honey-twice a day cures this problem in malnutritioned children.

(ii) Giving sweet mango is also useful.

Fever : —

Applying the paste of roots of mango on palms and soles of patient checks and cures fever.

Cholera : —

Taking decoction of fresh Mango leaves boiled in glass of water till it is reduced to half-twice a day helps in curing cholera.

Tuberculosis : —

Taking 1 cup sweet mango juice with 50 gms. of honey-twice a day regularly-helps in curing this.

Sun-Stroke : —

Taking raw mango's 'Panna' (Boil or roast a raw mango-mix in its pulp-Gur, roasted ground Jeera, Coriander, salt & powder of black-pepper & water) 3 or 4 times a day-eliminates the effect of sun-stroke.

Taking it daily in summers acts as a preventive against heat-stroke.

Fire Burn : —

(i) Applying the burnt ashes of mango leaves on the burnt part gives quick relief.

(ii) Applying the Mango Kernel got after rubbing on wet stone on the affected part also is useful.

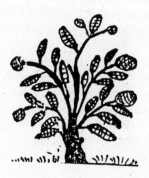

AMLA (Emblic Myrobalans)

1. Amla is known in different languages as : —

1.	Sanskrit	—	*Vayasya, Amalaki, Vrsya, Jatiphala-rasa, siva Dhatri-phala, Amrta, Amrtaphala.*
2.	Hindi	—	*Amla, Anvala,*
3.	Latin	—	*Phyllanthus*
4.	Bengali	—	*Amla, Amalaki*
5.	Marathi	—	*Kamavattha,*
6.	Gujarati	—	*Amla*
7.	Tamil	—	*Nellikai*
8.	Sindhi	—	*Amla*
9.	English	—	*Emblic Myrobalans.*

2. Description : —

Amla tree is found in all parts of India. It is generally 20-30 ft high. Its bark is rough and brownish in colour. It has irregular branches, bluish-yellow flowers, small leaves like that of tamarind. Its fruit is round and greenish yellow in colour with six segments with a hard seed inside. There are different varieties of this fruit of which Kalami, is the best for it has lot of pulp, very small seed and is comparatively less sour and bitter in taste than others. Kalami Amla is generally used in making Murabba, Chyavanprasha etc.

Hindus consider Amla tree as very sacred. It is believed that having food under Amla tree on 'Akshya Navami' in month of Kartika-leads to longevity. Amla is unique in this that-the fruit does not leave its chemical ingredients even when heated on fire. Every single part of the fruit-rind, pulp, seed etc. is used for medicinal purposes. Moreover, Amla tree purifies the air and atmosphere.

Amla is sour and bitter in taste. It controls imbalances caused by Vat (wind), Pitta (Bile) and kaph (Phlegm.) and is very effective in controlling digestive problems. It strengthens cardiac muscles, invigorates physical and mental faculties, improves eyesight, imparts natural glow and lustre to the body and hair. It is very useful in diarrhoea and is diuretic in nature. Its regular intake leads to healthy long life.

3. Chemical Properties : —

Amla is a rich source of "Vitamin C", which is 4 times more than an orange or eight times more than a tomato. Intake of $1\frac{1}{2}$ oz. juice of Amla everyday fulfils the daily human requirement of Vitamin 'C' which is about 50 mg.

Apart from this it has Gallic Acid, Tannic Acid, Sugar, Albumen, Calcium, Proteins, Phosphorus, Carbo-hydrates, Iron etc.

4. Curative Properties Of Amla : —

General Tonic : —

(i) Taking one raw Amla everyday in the morning removes general weakness of the different parts of the body.

(ii) Taking milk in the morning after licking one teaspoon of ground Amla powder mixed with honey-imparts freshness & strength to the body.

(iii) Taking the pulp of fresh Amla or Amla juice with honey or ghee in morning and evening-sharpens the intellect and invigorates the body.

(iv) Taking Amla and Black Til (in equal quantity) with honey or ghee cures mental and physical weakness.

(v) Taking one piece of Amla murabba with a cup of plain milk (without-Sugar) regularly for few days-cures general weakness and strengthens weakened brain.

Eye ailments : —

(i) Taking Amla daily in the morning or 1 tsp. Amla powder with water at night improves eye-sight.

(ii) Washing the eyes with Amla water (Soak Amla in water at night and strain it) in the morning-keeps eyes fresh, sparkling and improves eye-sight.

(iii) Washing the eyes with ground Amla and Til powder water (Soak Amla and Til powder in water over night and strain it) in the morning-cures burning sensation in the eyes.

(iv) Applying pulp of Amla on the head and washing the hair after massage-helps in curing burning sensation in the eyes and heaviness of the head.

(v) Taking Amla powder with milk cures ailment of the eyes-like sight loss or cataract.

(vi) Washing the eyes with water having triphala powder cures trachoma and other ailments of the eyes.

(vii) Eating 10 gms. of Triphala powder with 1 tsp. of honey everyday-keeps eyes very healthy strong and sparkling.

(viii) Taking 1 tsp. Triphala Powder (Harar, Bahed and Amla) mixed with half teaspoon of Pure ghee-everyday in the morning-improves eye-sight and cures weakness of the eyes or darkness coming before eyes.

Heart And Mental Weakness And Ailments : —

(i) Taking Amla Murabba everyday in the morning cures physical and mental debility.

(ii) Taking fresh juice of Amla mixed with water (in between- taking of food) removes weakness of body, mind and heart.

(iii) Massaging the scalp with Amla oil before going to bed-removes mental weakness.

(iv) Taking Amla powder with cow's milk or Mishri (same quantity) with water gives relief in heart ailments.

(v) Taking Amla Murabba everyday strengthens mental faculties and sharpens memory.

(vi) Applying paste made up of dried Amla powder with Kumkum, Neelkamal and Gulabjal cures headache.

(vii) Applying paste of juice of 2 or 3 Amla or its pulp mixed with little rose-water and 3 or 4 pieces of Kesar in it-on affected part for 15-minutes relieves the pain of migraine.

Night-discharge : —

(i) Taking 10 gm. fresh Amla juice with 1 gm. powdered Haldi and honey morning and evening regularly cures night discharge.

(ii) Taking Amla water (Soak dried Amla powder in 1 :3 proportion in water for 12 hours, strain the water and mix 1 gm. Haldi powder) regularly helps in curing night discharge.

Urinary Problems : —

(i) Taking 1 gm. Amla powder, Kalajeera and 2 gm. ground mishri with cold water-cures the habit of urinating in the bed at night.

(ii) Taking milk after eating fresh Amla juice or dried Amla powder with Gur-cures strangury.

(iii) Applying paste of Amla near the navel portion-helps in curing urinary problems.

(iv) Boil 20 gm. pulp of dried Amla in 160 gm. water till 40 gms. is left. Then mix 20 gm. Gur in it Drinking this helps in urinary problems.

(v) Taking crushed Amla pulp (after straining it) mixed with mishri cures blood in urine.

(vi) Taking 20 gm. fresh Amla juice with 10 gm. honey and water twice a day cures urinating problems.

Acidity : —

Licking one teaspoon of dried Amla powder with honey or ghee after dinner checks acidity.

Leucorrhoea : —

(i) Taking 3 gm. powdered Amla with 6 gm. honey everyday for one month cures this.

(ii) Taking-powder of Amla seed with honey or mishri-regularly helps in curing it.

(iii) Taking 20 gm. fresh Amla juice mixed with honey-regularly for a month checks leucorrhoea.

Blood-impurities : —

(i) Taking fresh Amla juice or Amla powder in tablet form-checks impurities of blood.

(ii) Taking 5 gms. of powder (made from 20 gms. Triphala, 20 gms. black pepper, 10 gms. pure sulphur, 5 gms. of Neem leaves and Mehandi leaves-ground in fine powder form) with a glass of water twice a day-cures all impurities in blood.

Diabetes : —

Taking fresh Amla juice with honey checks diabetes.

Piles : —

(i) Soak 15 gms. Amla and 15 gm. Mehndi leaves in 400 gm. water overnight Strain it . Drinking this water checks piles.

(ii) Taking 5 gm. of Triphala churna with a glass of whey-helps in curing piles.

(iii) Taking fresh Amla juice with $\frac{1}{2}$ tsp. ghee, 1 tsp. honey and 100 gm. of milk-after lunch cures- chronic piles.

Stone in Urinary Bladder : —

Taking Amla powder with radish helps in checking stone in bladder, breaking the stones and throwing it out with urine.

Diarrhoea : —

(i) Taking fresh Amla leaves with whey cures loose motions due to indigestion.

(ii) Taking juice of 5 fresh Amlas with glucose or grape juice-checks diarrhoea.

(iii) Rubbing the juice of Amala on the gums of child-helps in checking loose motions due to teething problem.

(iv) Swallowing dried Amla powder and Kaala Namak (equal quantity) with water cures loose motions.

Dysentery : —

Taking 20 gms. of fresh Amla juice with 5 gms. honey and 100 gms. of milk-3 or 4 times a day helps in curing dysentery.

Constipation : —

(i) Taking 1 tsp. dried Amla powder with milk or water before sleep at night helps in discharging bowels easily.

(ii) Taking strained water of meshed fresh Amlas soaked overnight in lukewarm water, helps in evacuating the bowels.

(iii) Taking 4 tsp. fresh Amla juice and 3 tsp. honey mixed in a glass of water-relieves constipation.

Worms : —

Taking about 20 gm. fresh Amla juice daily-kills worms.

Cough and Cold : —

(i) Taking two tsp. of fresh Amla juice with honey twice a day- helps in taking out the phlegm. and controls cold.

(ii) Taking milk in which a little Amla powder and ghee is boiled in the evening-helps in dry cough.

(iii) Licking Amla powder with honey-regularly twice or thrice a day-cures chronic dry cough.

Chronic Fever : —

Eating Mung Ki Dal with dried Amla powder cooked in it controls chronic fever.

Dryness in the body : —

Taking tea boiled with pieces of Amla in it mixed with sugar and milk cures dryness of skin.

Itching : —

Applying Amla churna in chameli oil (Dry Amlas in shade, powder them and mix in chameli oil. The bottle should be kept in shade) on the part of the body where itching is there- gives relief.

Baldness : —

Washing the head with Amla-juice mixed water after rubbing the scalp for 10-15 minutes with fresh Amla juice-helps in growing of hair.

Cuts : —

Applying fresh Amla juice on the wound caused by the cut-stops bleeding and is an antiseptic.

High blood-pressure : —

Taking juice of fresh Amla or Murabba Amla everyday in the morning controls high blood-pressure.

Anaemia : —

Taking $\frac{1}{2}$ cup Amla juice, 2 tsp. honey with little water-regularly helps in curing anaemia.

Stammering : —

Taking one raw fresh Amla everyday relieves stammering in children.

Nose-bleeding : —

(i) Taking Amla Ka Murabba everyday helps in curing bleeding of nose.

(ii) Washing the hair with water in which dried Amlas have been soaked overnight-gives relief.

(iii) Putting drop of fresh Amla juice in the nostril or smelling the juice or applying the paste of Amla on the forehead helps in checking the flow of blood.

Thirst due to dehydration : —

Taking Amla juice with grape juice or honey in the form of sharbat-quenches thirst & cures dehydration caused by diarrhoea, dysentery.

Hair-loss and other problems : —

(i) Soak dried Amla, Harer, Baher and Shikakai in an iron utensil overnight Mesh them nicely. Washing regularly with this strengthens the hair, imparts glow and lustre, smoothness and blackness and also stops excessive hair-fall.

(ii) Applying the paste of dried Amla and Mehandi leaves on the hair 10 or 15 minutes before washing-make the hair black and strong.

(iii) Applying the paste of Amla powder mixed in lemon-juice on the hair 10 or 15 minutes before washing with Amla water-keeps- the hair strong and shining.

(iv) Washing the hair with decoction of Amla-removes dryness of the scalp, checks dandruff and stops excessive fall and greying of hair.

(v) Massaging the head with Amla oil imparts natural glow to hair, relieves mental tensions and induces sleep.

Jaundice : —

(i) Soak 4 Munakkas in juice of 4 fresh Amla. After one hour grind the soaked munakkas and mix it with Amla juice taking this twice a day gives relief in Jaundice.

(ii) Taking and licking little churna (made by grinding 10 gms. each of Amla, dry ginger, black pepper, 3 gm. of Iron Bhasm and little turmeric-) with honey-cures Jaundice.

Digestive Problems : —

(i) Taking 10 gms. fresh Amla juice with 10 gms. pomegranate juice, 20 gm. Jaggery and 2 ground cloves-(a) early in the morning before breakfast and (b) after food-cures constipation, wind-problems, other effects of indigestion.

(ii) Taking two tsp. of fresh Amla juice mixed with two tsp. sugar or 2 tsp. dried Amla powder mixed with same amount of Mishri with water cures this.

(iii) Taking Amla juice morning and evening-cures chronic indigestion.

(iv) Eating raw Amla on empty stomach everyday is very useful for the digestive system.

(v) Taking dried Amla powder and little Kaala Namak with lukewarm water in summer and with honey in winter after meals cures all digestive problems.

Gout : —

Taking fresh Amla juice with old ghee-heated a little-regularly for few days-relieves stiffness of joints and helps in curing Gout.

Itching, Burning-after Measles Chicken Pox, Small Pox : —

(i) Taking bath with water having fresh Amla juice in it or having Amlas boiled in it-relieves the itching and burning sensation after measles or chicken pox.

(ii) Apply the paste made of Amla and Til in equal quantity ground in cold milk added with 3 or 4 drops of rose water on spots and let it stay for sometime and then wash. This helps in removing the spots.

Boils in Mouth : —

Doing gargles with water having fresh Amla juice-twice or thrice a day gives relief. After gargles-apply fresh Amla juice on the boils and let saliva ooze out.

Giddiness, darkness before eyes : —

(i) Taking fresh Amla juice with honey in the morning-cures this.

(ii) Taking Harar, Bahar and Amla Churna (Triphala) in one tsp. mixed with $\frac{1}{2}$ tsp. of pure ghee-in the morning helps in improvement of eye-sight and curing of giddiness, darkness etc.

(iii) Licking one tsp. of powdered Amla with 1 tsp. of honey- morning and evening-gives strength to the body and cures darkness before eyes.

Lices in hair :—

Applying the paste of ground seeds of Amla mixed with juice of lemon-on the roots of the hair, and washing after half an hour will clear the lices.

Obesity :—

Drinking a glass of Amla water (in which Amlas have been soaked overnight) with 1 tsp. of honey-early in the morning-helps in slimming.

Menstrual Disorder :—

(i) Taking boiled pulp of Amla with honey two times a day- relieves one of very scanty and painful bleeding.

(ii) Taking Amla juice mixed with ripe banana 3 or 4 times a day during periods-checks profuse bleeding.

Insect-bite :—

(i) Applying the paste made of triphala powder mixed with cow's urine-on the affected part-relieves the poisonous effect of insects.

(ii) Drinking of Amla juice is also very helpful.

Beauty-treatment :—

(i) Applying paste of Amla mixed with turmeric and oil-on the body-makes the skin clear, soft and improves the complexion..

(ii) Drinking Amla juice (Amlas to be soaked overnight-crushed and then strained) mixed with honey-in the morning-makes the complexion full of natural glow and charm.

(iii) Applying the paste of soaked wet seeds of Amla on the face-eliminates pimples and gives natural beauty.

We find that Amla is one of the important ingredients of 'Triphala' (i.e. Harar, Bahad and Amla) out of which many Ayurved drugs are made. It is really a rich storehouse of medicinal properties, helpful in eliminating and curing various physical and mental weakness and ailments. Apart from this use- Amla can also be used as food-item in different forms :—

(i) Munching raw Amla or one piece of Amla Murabba followed by milk-is an ideal breakfast for persons of all age-groups.

(ii) Taking chutney or pickle of Amla with meals is invigorating and digestive.

(iii) Taking Chyavanaprash in the morning with milk is the best tonic for one and all.

(iv) Taking sharbat of Amla especially in summer is refreshing and is a tonic.

Amla, undoubtedly, is capable of imparting glow and lustre and physical, mental strength and vigour to different parts of the body and also eliminating various diseases. It is an efficacious and extremely cheap 'Amrit Phala', which could be used by rich and poor alike for healthy long life.

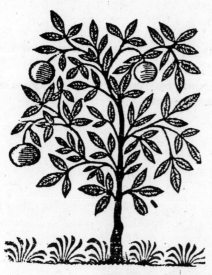
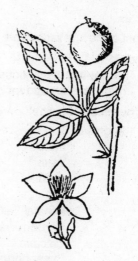

BAEL(Bangal Kins)

1. Bael is known in different languages as : —

1.	Sanskrit	—	*Bilva, Shriphala, Malur*
2.	Hindi	—	*Bel, Shivphala, Sriphala*
3.	Latin	—	*Aegle Marmelos*
4.	Bengali	—	*Bilva, Bel*
5.	Marathi	—	*Belvriksha, Belphala*
6.	Kannada	—	*Bellu*
7.	Telegu	—	*Matidi*
8.	Gujrati	—	*Beelee, Villovidhu*
9.	Sindhi	—	*Bel*
10.	English	—	*Bangal Kins*

2. Description : —

Bael tree is a very sacred tree. Its leaves and flowers are offered to Lord Siva by Hindus in temples. Its wood is considered very pure and is used for performing sacrifices.

Bael tree is a big tree-30 to 40 ft in height, with a thick trunk without any thorns. But its branches are thin, sharp, strong and thorny. The tree starts flowering in winter and gives ripe fruits in summer. The unripe fruit has a soft green covering with greenish yellow pulp in it, where as the ripe fruit has a very hard yellow coloured outer covering with reddish yellow pulp in it. The weight of the fruit varies from 100 gms to $2\frac{1}{2}$ kg. This tree is found everywhere in India.

The ripe-fruit is nutritious, delicious, aromatic and laxative and both ripe and un-ripe fruit is used for curing many ailments.

3. Chemical Composition of Bael : —

100 gms of Bael consists of

Food	—	64 gms.
Water	—	61.5 gms
Protein	—	1.8
Fat	—	0.3
Mineral Salts	—	1.7
Carbohydrates	—	31.8
Calcium	—	85 mg
Phosphorus	—	50 gm
Iron	—	0.6
Calories	—	137

Apart from this Bael has 55 mg Karotin, 0.92 mg-Vitamin Bi. 1.19-Vitamin B, 1-mg-Nycin and 8 mg-Vitamin C.

Bael is a rich store of tannic acid. Its pulp contains mucilage pectin, tannin, volatile oil, bitter principle and ash 2% and Sugar also.

The outer shell contains potassium and sodium compounds, lime and iron phosphates, magnesium, calcium carbonate, silica etc.

The leaves on distillation yield yellowish-green-coloured oil, which has aromatic odour and bitter taste.

4. Curative properties of Bael : —

Diarrhoea and dysentery : —

(i) Pulp of unripe Bael with Chacha (Whey) controls Diarrhoea.

(ii) Pulp of ripe Bael with water checks Diarrhoea.

(iii) Preparation made by boiling pulp of unripe or half ripe Bael fruit acts as an anti-flatulent and controls acidity, Diarrhoea. and dysentery.

(iv) Murabba of bael also helps in controlling Diarrhoea. and dysentery.

(v) Decoction of unripe Bael fruit baked for 6 hrs. with Mishri controls dysentery.

Dyspepsia : —

Syrup of ripe fruit helps in dyspepsia.

Piles : —

Pulp of Ripe fruit mixed with Mishri checks constipation and controls piles.

Vomiting : —

(i) Decoction of unripe Bael fruit controls vomiting.

(ii) Pulp of ripe fruit (20 gms) mixed with water of boiled rice and little mishri-controls vomiting during pregnancy.

Anaemia : —

(i) 5 gms Powder of dried pulp mixed with milk & little sugar checks anaemia.

(ii) Powder of dried pulp with Chacha (whey) with little sugar eliminates blood-impurities.

Leucorrhoea : —

Make powder of 10 gm pulp of Bael, mixed with 10 gm Nagkesar and 10 gr-Rasont.

5 gms of this mixture taken with Maand (boiled-rice water)-checks leucorrhoea.

Teething : —

Boil 10 gms powdered dried pulp of Bael fruit in 150 gms. water till the quantity of water is 20 gms.

5 gms-of this mixed with little honey administered thrice a day for 3 days helps in teething.

Uses Of Leaves Of Bael : —

Cholera : —

50 Gms juice of leaves mixed with little lemon-juice and Desi Khand-taken daily-prevents Cholera.

Whooping Cough : —

Roast the green leaves on slow fire till they become black Powder. Filter them through cloth, 1 or 2 gms of this powder taken with little honey 3 times a day checks whooping cough.

Kanthamala : —

Make a paste of fresh leaves mixed with pure ghee. Apply the paste twice a day around the neck and cover with a cloth. It helps in eliminating Kanthamala.

Night blindness (Nyctalopia) : —

Grind 10 gms fresh leaves and 7 seeds of black pepper with little water and mix it with 25 gms of sugar in 100 gms water. Taking this twice a day helps in night-blindness.

Also soak a few leaves in water overnight and wash the eyes with that in the morning.

Bronchites : —

Poultice prepared from the leaves is applied to the chest in acute bronchitis.

Asthma :—

A decoction of leaves of Bael helps in asthma.

Diabetes :—

(i) Juice of Bael leaves with ground black pepper is useful in Diabetes.

(ii) Chewing 4-6 Bael-leaves daily controls sugar.

Urinary Irritation :—

Juice of Bael-leaves, ground Jeera and Mishri (all in equal quantity) taken with milk stops urinary irritation.

Repellant of mosquitoes and insects :—

Burning of outershell of the Bael-repels all insects and mosquitos.

Thus the Bael tree is very significant. Apart from nutritional and medicinal value of the ripe, and unripe fruit-pulp the other parts of the tree-its bark, flowers, leaves, trunk etc. have their special properties and uses. Bael is widely used as a medicine in households.

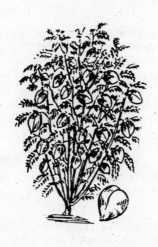

CHANA (Gram)

1. Chana is known in different languages as : —

1.	Sanskrit	—	*Chanaka, Harimanthaka, Sakal-priya, Yechana*
2.	Hindi	—	*Chana, Boota*
3.	Latin	—	*Cicer Arietinum*
4.	Bengali	—	*Chola*
5.	Marathi	—	*Chande*
6.	Kannada	—	*Kadale*
7.	Gujrati	—	*Chana*
8.	Sindhi	—	*Chana*
9.	English	—	*Gram*

2. Description : —

Chana is very popular throughout India and is one of the staple cereals taken in North India. It is eaten in all the stages of its growth. The tiny tender leaves of chana known as Chana Ka Saag, (eaten raw and also cooked as vegetable); green grains known as Hola (eaten after roasting near Holi), ripe grains as (chana flour without husk) and ground Atta (mixed with or without wheat flour) and many other tasty delicious preparations are made from chana.

It is very nutritive. Regular intake of Chana imparts a lot of physical vigour and strength to the muscles and all parts of the body.

Chana is invigorating, purifier of blood, digestive, antibilleous and anti phlegm.atic, anti pyreutic, pain-killer, germicidal, and very effective in cold and cough.

3. Chemical Properties :—

Chana is very rich source of Protein. The leaves of Chana contain lots of Vitamin 'A'. The sprouted chanas are full of Vitamin C, B and E.

Note :—

(i) Chana should be taken along with its husk for that helps in assimilating full protein in the body.

(ii) Excessive intake of Besan should be avoided as it causes indigestion and diarrhoea.

(iii) Water should not be taken just after eating chanas, chapatis, puri etc. for the gram flour will form a paste with water and that will cause constipation and indigestion.

Curative Properties of Chana :—

General Tonic :—

(i) Sprouted Chanas (Soak chanas for 1 day in summers & 2 days in winters. Hang them for 2 days in a wet cloth and they are sprouted) with grated ginger, little sendha Namak, Black pepper and lemon-juice sprinkled on it is an ideal breakfast. This is very rich in Vitamin C and gives strength and energy to the entire body.

(ii) Taking 200 gms. milk (in which 20 gms. of chana or 40 gms. of chane ki dal had been soaked over night) in the breakfast after chewing finely the soaked chanas or chane ki dal-gives lot of stamina.

(iii) Taking Chutney of green gram-strengthens bones and muscles of the body.

(iv) Taking chanas regularly makes the man's muscles very strong and free from problems like early ejaculation or lack of sexual power.

Anaemia :—

Taking sprouted chanas in breakfast cures anaemia.

Arthritis :—

Taking boiled grams with honey in the morning makes the joints supple.

Heart trouble :—

Taking roasted Chana or soaked black Chana is very useful for heart patients.

Indigestion and stomach problem :—

(i) Taking sprouted Chana in the morning stimulates appetite.

(ii) Taking Raita of Bundi (made from ground gram) with little roasted Jeerapowder, dry Pudina powder with food eliminates all digestive problems.

(iii) Taking 10-15 gms. juice of soft fresh leaves of Chana plant eliminates gases.

Constipation : –

Eating Chana (soaked overnight) in the morning with ground Jeera and Sonth sprinkled on it and also drinking the water (in which Chana was soaked) eliminates constipation.

Cold : –

(i) Taking milk after eating roasted chana before going to bed- eliminates the phlegm. and clears the wind pipe.

(ii) Smelling the roasted hot-chana (tied in a potli) stops running nose.

(iii) Eating roasted chanas helps in releasing trapped phlegm..

(iv) Eating thick chapati of chana choker flour with little Ajwain, Heeng, black-pepper powder-cooked on slow fire with thin dal helps in curing chronic cold.

Stones : –

(i) Taking Chana ki Dal Soaked overnight with honey helps in breaking the stones in bladder, kidney and throwing them out.

(ii) Drinking water of Black Chana and wheat (which have been soaked overnight and boiled in the morning) is also very useful.

(iii) Eating chapatis made of ground chana and wheat regularly is useful in dissolving and throwing out of stones.

Asthma : –

(i) Taking 40-50 gms. of roasted chanas in the evening-followed with hot milk-clears the phlegm. in the bronchial chords.

(ii) Eating whole gram Parantha or Rotis with pieces of onion stuffed in it followed by hot milk eliminates excessive phlegm. in the respiratory system.

Hoarse Voice : –

Eating crushed black chana (soaked over night) boiled in 250 gms. milk with 2 tsp. of honey-slowly helps in de-straining the vocal- chords and cures hoarse voice.

Skin-Care : –

(i) Washing the face with ground chana (Besan)-removes spots and freckles.

(ii) Applying the paste of Besan with mustard oil-on the affected part softly and gradually rubbing it off the skin after 30-40 minutes-clears the skin, improves the complexion, removes the white patches (especially if they are due to dryness in winter season).

(iii) Applying a paste of Besan with milk or curd-on the face for half an hour-improves the complexion and imparts glow.

Hair :—

Applying a solution of Besan with water on the hair for 10-15 minutes and then washing with lukewarm water eliminates dryness of the hair, makes them soft and lustrous and checks dandruff.

Itching skin ailments :—

(i) Eating ground .chana roti without salt, with or without ghee regularly-for 2 months eliminates blood impurities, itching and cures all skin problems.

(ii) Taking sprouted Gram early in the morning and also the water in which they were soaked-eliminates all blood impurities.

(iii) Applying a smooth paste of Gram plant mixed with mustard oil on the body half an hour before bath-eliminates itching sensation of the body.

(iv) Taking chutney made of Gramplant purifies the skin and gives energy.

Leucoderma :—

(i) Eating ground chana chapati is very useful.

(ii) Sprouted chanas (Soak 20 gm. chana with 10 gm. of Triphala Harar, Bahar, Amla-in 125 gm. water and then keep it for 24 hours for sprouting) regularly helps in curing leucoderma.

Urticaria :—

(i) Eating Besan Laddus with black-pepper sprinkled on it-cures urticaria.

(ii) Taking Besan Bundi Raita with black-pepper and sugar-cures urticaria.

Pain :—

Massaging the affected part of the body with Besan eliminates pain.

Vomitting :—

(i) Taking water only in which chana has been soaked, helps in curing vomiting.

(ii) Taking Sattu of chana with water and sugar (Sattu by grinding roasted gram and barley) controls vomiting during pregnancy.

Diarrhoea :—

Taking the water of chana husk (Soaked for half an hour. keep it on cloth and have the oozed out water) frequently stops loose motions.

Leucorrhoea :—

Eating ground roasted chana with jaggery followed by drinking milk with pure ghee-helps in curing leucorrhoea.

Piles :—

Eating slightly hot roasted chana helps in curing piles.

Jaundice :—

Taking chana ki dal soaked overnight with Gur in equal quantity for 3-4 days and also drinking the same water (in which Dal was soaked) when thirsty-helps in eliminating jaundice.

Polyuria :—

(i) Taking little Gur after eating 10 gm. roasted chanas-regularly checks tendency of frequent urinating.

(ii) Roasted chana taken without water also checks polyuria.

Abortion,-Delivery etc. :—

(i) Taking decoction of Black Chana (by boiling 200 gms. chana in 400 gms. water till the water is reduced to half) regularly after conception is preventive against abortion.

(ii) Taking 10 gms. barley gram ground powder with little ground Black Til and Sugar followed by a glass of hot milk-after the conception regularly-is also very useful to prevent abortion.

(iii) Chapatis made of ground wholegram and moth (a variety of pulse) with lunch and dinner-cleans the insides of the ovaries after delivery or abortion.

Increase in mother's milk :—

(i) Taking the boiled milk (in which Kabuli Chana has been soaked overnight) after chewing the chanas regularly helps the mother to have adequate milk in the breasts.

(ii) Chana (with husk) with honey or sugar also is useful.

Diabetes :—

(i) Taking Black Chana (soaked in milk overnight) eliminates sugar.

(ii) Chapatis of ground Gram mixed with ground barley of only Besan in lunch and dinner cures diabetes.

Worms :—

Taking Chana soaked overnight in vinegar in breakfast with little salt and onion pieces throws the worms out. (Caution-any amount of water can be taken but nothing solid in breakfast and lunch).

Semen :—

(i) Taking roasted chana or soaked chana with almonds (in the same proportion) followed by drinking milk, thickens the semen.

(ii) Soaked chane ki dal in the morning and at night with or without sugarcandy strengthens and enhances sexual potency.

Eye-Trouble : —

(i) Eating freshly roasted chana or soaked chanas gives relief to the tired and swollen eyes.

(ii) Taking fresh leaves of the Chana plant-is good for enhancing eye-sight.

(iii) Chane-ka-Saag with butter is also good for eyes.

(iv) Binding the freshly roasted chana in a potli-to foment the eyes and putting drop of rose-water reduces redness, pain and burning sensation in the eyes.

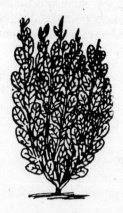

DHANIA (Coriander Seed)

1. Dhania Is Known In Different Languages As : —

1.	Sanskrit	—	*Dhanyaka, Dhanya, Dhenuka, Dhanaka, Vitunnaka,*
2.	Hindi	—	*Dhania*
3.	Latin	—	*Coriandrum sativum*
4.	Bengali	—	*Dhanne*
5.	Marathi	—	*Dhane*
6.	Kannada	—	*Konthavuri*
7.	Telegu	—	*Konthamelu*
8.	Gujrati	—	*Dhana*
9.	Tamil	—	*Kotamalli*
10.	Sindhi	—	*Dhania*
11.	English	—	*Coriander Seed.*

2. Description : —

Dhania is very popular and grown all over India. The plant is small with tiny branches, which bear leaves and inflorescence. These flowers turn into small sized, round shaped seeds having two segments, and are known as Dhania.

Fresh leaves (as flavouring agent) and dried Dhania seeds (as spices) are used in curries, chutney etc. Dhania has aromatic oil and is slightly pungent.

This is a great flavouring agent, stimulant, carminative, helps in stomach ache and griping pain, tranquiliser, germicidal, diuretic, anti-pyretic, curtails excessive requirement of water in digestive system and is a tonic.

3. Composition :–

Water	84%
Volatile oil	1%
Fixed oil	13%
Mucilage	3%
Tannin, Malic acid & Ash	5%

Curative Properties Of Dhania :–

Asthma, cough (dry) :–

(i) Taking 1 tsp of Dhania powder and mishri in boiled rice-water 3 times a day controls cough.

(ii) 1 tsp Dhania sharbat mixed with 1 tsp honey 3 times a day cures dry cough (Soak 50 gm coarsely ground Dhania in 500 gm. water overnight. Boil till decoction is 125 gms. Strain it through cloth and prepare (chashni) sharbat with 250 gm Desi sugar).

Frequent Sneezing :–

Smelling fresh coriander leaves stops sneezing.

Diarrhoea, Indigestion :–

(i) 1 tsp of Dhania Churn (10 gms Dhania, 10 gms Illayachi & 10 gms Jeera-fried and powdered) after meals controls diarrhoea, cures indigestion and increases appetite.

(ii) 1 tsp of heated powdered Dhania with water checks loose motions.

(iii) 5 gms heated powdered Dhania with curd or skimmed curd or water every 4 hours is useful.

(iv) $\frac{1}{2}$ tsp Dhania powder with little Kala Namak after meals helps.

(v) $\frac{1}{2}$ tsp of mixture (60 gm dry Dhania powder 25 gm black pepper and 25 gm salt) with water after meals cures tendency to go to toilet after meals.

Dysentery :–

1 tsp of decoction of Dhania powder and Mishri (10 gm s each) 3 times a day-cures dysentery.

Wind :–

(i) 1 tsp Dried Dhania powder boiled in $\frac{1}{2}$ cup water-taken twice a day controls gaseous problems.

(ii) Oil of Dhania is carminative and used in flatulent colic.

Loss of Appetite :–

(i) Taking 30 gm juice of fresh Dhania leaves daily increases appetite.

(ii) 1 tsp of ground powder (Dhania, small Illayachi and black pepper in equal quantity) mixed with 1 tsp ghee and sugar eliminates dyspepsia.

Giddiness, Vomitting, Nausea : −

Dhania boiled in water mixed with Mishri eliminates nausea, giddiness and vomitting in pregnancy.

Headache : −

Applying juice of fresh Dhania leaves on forehead cures headache.

Mental Weakness : −

Boil 125 gm ground Dhania in 500 gm water till 125 gm remains. Then mix 125 gms Mishri in it till it gets thick. Taking it regularly cures mental weakness.

Throat-ache : −

(i) Chewing 1 gm Dhania seeds slowly 3 or 4 times a day or

(ii) 1 tsp of Dhania with 1 tsp of Mishri-4 times a day relieves throat-ache.

Stomach-ache : −

2 tsp Dhania Sharbat or 2 tsp Dhania boiled in 1 cup of water- taken 2 or 3 times relieves ache.

Malaria : −

$\frac{1}{2}$ tsp of Dhania powder with $\frac{1}{2}$ tsp sonth 3 times a day cures fever.

Heat stroke : −

Soak 100 gms ground Dhania in 500 gms water for 1 hour in a new earthen pot. Strain it and take $\frac{1}{2}$ cup water with 5 Batashas-every 3 hours. It cures giddiness, vomitting, nausea due to heat.

(ii) 1 tsp Dhania soaked in 1 cup water with sugar acts as preventive against heat stroke.

Blisters in mouth : −

(i) Applying ground Dhania or juice of fresh leaves on blisters cures them.

(ii) Gargle with Dhania boiled water cures blisters.

Kanthamala : −

(i) Paste of Dhania and barley flour in equal quantity or

(ii) Paste of fresh Dhania leaves with gram flour and Gulab Jal- applied daily cures Kanthamala.

Bite of Poisonous Insects : −

Taking some Dhania seeds with cold water and applying fresh Dhania juice mixed with vinegar relieves the stinging sensation.

Night-discharge : —

(i) Taking 4 gm powdered Dhania mixed with Mishri with fresh water in the morning for 7 days cures night-discharge or

(ii) 1 tsp of fresh Dhania paste with Mishri and cold water in the morning or

(iii) 1 tsp. of powdered Dhania and sugar with water in the morning and evening prevents night-discharge, or

(Note : Don't eat any thing for 1 hour after this dose.)

(iv) Dhania powder mixed with Mishri in cold water taken before sleep cures this.

Baldness : —

Applying juice of fresh leaves on the head-makes hair grow.

Piles : —

Dhania juice with Mishri cures blood oozing from piles.

2 tsp Dhania (fried in little ghee) & 2 tsp sugar boiled in 500 gms milk taken hot in place of tea or coffee for sometimes cures piles.

Eyesight : —

Taking 1 tsp of paste of Dhania leaves or 1 tsp Dhania mixed with Amla improves eyesight.

Insomnia : —

(i) Paste of Coriander leaves with sugar to taste taken in water induces sleep.

(ii) Application of juice of fresh leaves on forehead is also useful.

(iii) 20 or 30 gm sharbat (by boiling fresh Dhania leaves and Mishri in same quantity) daily induces sleep.

(iv) 3 to 5 gms of powder with Gulabjal (made by mixing powdered Dhania, Khaskhas, Binole seeds 10 gms each with 20 gms Khand).

Menstrual Disorders : —

(i) Dhania powder with boiled rice water checks excessive bleeding during menses.

(ii) Boil 20 gm Dhania in 200 gm water till the water is 50 gm. Taking the mixture with Mishri checks excessive bleeding.

Strangury : —

Soak 30 gm half ground Dhania in 500 gm boiling water in an earthern pot overnight. After straining it in the morning mix 30 gm Batasha.

8-10 gms of this taken 4-5 times in a day for sometime cures strangury.

BLEEDING through Nose : —

(i) Applying paste of fresh leaves on forehead and smelling juice of fresh leaves stops nose-bleeding due to heat.

(ii) Taking paste of Dhania (soaked overnight) in the morning is also useful.

General tonic : —

Juice of 100 gms fresh Dhania leaves, taken daily is a source of all vitamins.

Note : — Fresh Dhania leaves, as flavouring agent, should be used in raw form to present loss of Vitamins caused by heating or boiling.

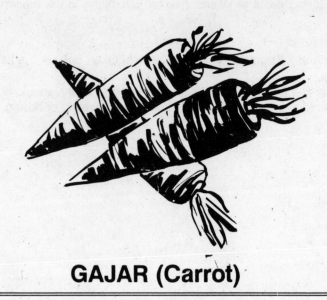

GAJAR (Carrot)

1. Carrot is known in different languages as :—

1.	Hindi	—	*Gajar*
2.	Latin	—	*Docks Carota*
3.	Gujrati	—	*Gajar*
4.	Sindhi	—	*Gajar*
5.	English	—	*Carrot*

2. Description :—

Carrot is grown all over India and is available in large quantities between October to March. It is of varied colours- black, pinkish red, and yellow. Carrot because of its great nutritive value is used as fruit and vegetable. It is within the reach of rich and poor alike and is rightly called "Apple of the poor". Its root is the main edible part. It is taken raw as salad juice, and cooked as vegetable, jam, Murabba, Kheer, Raita, Sharbat and many other varieties.

Carrots maintain acidic and alkaline proportion in the system. It is an invigorating and energy giving tonic for eyes, skin, bones, heart and muscles of the body. It is blood-purifier, diuretic, carminative, digestive, antiflatulent, antipyreutic and vermifuge. (Note : Persons suffering from dysentery or wounds in the intestines should not eat 'raw' carrots.)

3. Chemical Properties of Carrot : —

Carrot is rich source of carotine, Vitamin A, B, C, Iron, Calcium sugar, phosphorus etc. 100 gms. of Carrot contains the following : —

Water	-	86.0 gm.
Fat	-	0.2 gm.
Fibre	-	1.2 gm.
Calories	-	47.0 gm.
Calcium	-	80.0 mg.
Oxalic Acid	-	5.0 mg.
Protein	-	0.9 gm.
Minerals	-	1.1 gm.
Carbohydrates	-	10.6 gm.
Magnesium	-	14.0 mg.
Phosphorus	-	30.0 mg.
Iron	-	2.2 mg.
Potassium	-	108.0 mg.
Chlorine	-	0.13 mg.
Thiamine	-	0.04 mg.
Vitamin C	-	3.0 mg.
Sodium	-	35.6 mg.
Sulphur	-	27.0 mg.
Vitamin A	-	3.150 I.u.
Nicotine Acid	-	0.06 mg.

Its leaves contain water, Protein, Fats, Carbohydrates, Calcium, Phosphorus, Iron and Minerals.

4. Curative Properties of Carrot : —

General Tonic : —

(i) Eating raw Carrot or taking its juice is a very good tonic for eyes, skin, physical and mental development.

(ii) Giving 2-3 tsp. Carrot juice to weak children makes them physically strong.

Weak Memory : —

Taking Carrot juice with 2 cups of milk (preferably cow's milk) after eating 5-6 almonds early in the morning-sharpens memory.

Anaemia : —

(i) Taking slices of raw carrots and beetroot (Chukander) with lemon juice sprinkled on it-cures anaemia.

(ii) Taking 250 gms. juice of carrots with spinach juice-increases red-blood corpuscles.

Bleeding : —

Intake of carrots stops bleeding.

Nose bleeding : −

Applying paste of ground fresh carrot on forehead and above the nostrils-stops bleeding from nose. Drinking carrot juice is also advisable.

Headache : −

Taking juice of Carrot, beetroot and cucumber eliminates headache.

Migraine : −

Pouring a few drops of ghee-juice of soft leaves of carrot (Heat soft carrot leaves with ghee applied on it on fire and then extract the juice) in the ears and nostrils twice a day-induces sneezing and cures the disease.

Indigestion and stomach problems : −

(i) Taking juice of carrot and spinach after meals cures constipation and helps in easy bowel-movement.

(ii) Taking fresh carrots or its juice regularly cures indigestion, chronic diarrhoea, acidity and other stomach disorders.

(iii) Taking 200 gms. carrot juice mixed with 200 gms. curd (preferably made from goat's milk) in the morning-eliminates bleeding and cures amoebisis.

Cramps : −

Taking Halwa of grated red carrots (fried on fire with little ghee or butter and mixed with little jaggery) twice a day eliminates cramps and imparts strength.

Rheumatism : −

(i) Taking carrot juice regularly cures rheumatism.

(ii) Or carrot juice mixed with beetroot in equal quantity gives instant relief.

Arthrites : −

Taking 5 gms. carrot juice with $2\frac{1}{2}$ gms. of juice of Kanphool (Dandelion) regularly-makes the joint supple.

Gout : −

Taking carrot juice with parsley juice twice a day regularly reduces inflammation of the joints.

Eye-problems : −

(i) Taking carrot and spinach juice in equal proportion-improves eye-sight.

(ii) Taking fresh carrots or its juice daily is very good for eyes and cures even night-blindness.

(iii) Washing eyes with water in which carrots have been boiled- gives relief in case of eye-strain.

Asthma : –

Taking 1 cup of carrot juice mixed with $\frac{1}{2}$ cup of spinach juice regularly thrice a day gives relief in Asthma.

Obesity : –

Taking carrot juice mixed with lettuce juice-regularly eliminates extra fat.

Skin-troubles : –

(i) Taking raw carrots or its juice regularly eliminates aches, dryness of the skin, cures itching, removes blood-impurities and imparts natural glow.

(ii) Tying heated poultice of carrots on boils etc. cures them.

Eczema : –

(i) Taking carrot juice 3 times a day cures this, and

(ii) Also applying the pulp of carrots on the affected part eliminates the spots left by the disease.

Ringworm : –

Tying a hot poultice of grated carrot with sendha Namak sprinkled on the affected part cures the disease.

Fire-burn : –

Applying the crushed pulp of carrot on the affected part and taking its juice eliminates the burning sensation and cures it.

Tonsilitis : –

Taking carrot juice cures tonsilites.

Tooth Problems : –

Taking fresh carrots/1 cup carrot juice daily strengthens the gums and eliminates all dental problems.

Foul smell in mouth : –

Taking juice of carrots, spinach and cucumber in equal proportion-eliminates foul smell in mouth.

Blood-pressure : –

Taking carrot juice with spinach juice in 3 : 1 proportion regulates blood pressure.

Urinary problems : –

(i) Taking carrot juice regularly twice a day-keeps the urinary track clean and unobstructed.

(ii) Taking carrot juice and spinach juice (2 : 1 proportion) eliminates stranguary.

(iii) Taking 2 tsp. ground seeds of carrot boiled in 1 glass of water eliminates stranguary and cures other kidney problems.

Stone :—

(i) Taking 1 glass of juice of carrot, beetroot, cucumber (in equal proportion) helps in breaking stones and throwing them out.

(ii) Taking carrot juice 3 or 4 times a day is also useful.

(iii) Swallowing ground seeds of carrots with water also helps in this.

(iv) Taking 1 glass juice of carrot and lettuce (in equal quantity) eliminates stones from Gall Bladder.

Weak Heart :—

Taking carrot juice twice a day strengthens the heart.

Liver :—

Taking 1 cup fresh carrot juice with $\frac{1}{2}$ cup spinach juice everyday-cures liver problems. (*Notes :—* Gram flour is advised for the patients)

Jaundice :—

Taking fresh carrot juice or soup or hot decoction of carrots twice a day gives relief in jaundice.

Wound :—

Tying the pulp of boiled carrots on the wound heals the wounds. Carrot juice should also be taken.

Intestinal disorders :—

Taking juice of carrots, cabbage and tomatoes (in equal proportion) daily-cures all problems connected with intestines.

Worms :—

(i) Taking fresh carrot or any preparation of carrot regularly is helpful in expelling worms.

(ii) Taking 1 cup of carrot juice empty stomach regularly for 10-15 days helps in killing worms and extracting them out of the system.

(iii) Taking 1 glass Kanji of carrots regularly for 3-4 weeeks- expels the dead worms.

Pain in chest :—

Taking juice of boiled carrots with honey eliminates pain.

Spleen trouble :—

Taking pickle of carrots (soak pieces of carrots in water having powder of mustard seeds and little salt-for 2 to 3 days) with meals helps in curing spleen trouble.

Diabetes :—

(i) Taking carrot juice or carrot juice mixed with Karela juice daily in the morning helps in secretion of insulin in the body.

(ii) Taking carrot juice with spinach juice (2 :1 proportion) daily also is helpful.

Sexual weakness : –

(i) Taking carrot jam with milk 2 times a day eliminates weakness.

(ii) Taking carrot Kheer 2 times a day is also useful.

Lack of milk in breast : –

(i) Taking black carrots with milk (preferably right from cow's udder) brings enough milk for the child.

(ii) Taking juice of fresh carrots is also advisable.

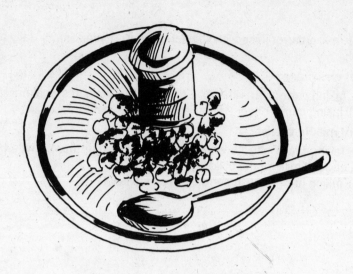

HEENG (Asafoetida)

1. Heeng is known in different languages as : —

1.	Sanskrit	—	*Jatuka, Hingu, Ramatha, Sahasravedhi, Vahlika*
2.	Hindhi	—	*Heeng*
3.	Latin	—	*Ferula foetida*
4.	Bengali	—	*Hingu*
5.	Marathi	—	*Hing*
6.	Telegu	—	*Ingura*
7.	Gujrati	—	*Hing*
8.	Sindhi	—	*Hing*
9.	English	—	*Asafoetida*

2. Description : —

Heeng is one of the most favourite and popular condiment used in preparing food, especially in Northern India. Heeng because of its nutritive qualities and efficacies, medicinal value and curative properties is a must in traditional houses in India.

Heeng is mainly of two different varieties based on the place of its origin (i) Chasha Vahlika-sown and produced in Balkh (ii) Ramatha-in Afghanistan or India.

Heeng's plant has lot of leaves and comes to us after refinement. Cut is made in the plant just below the stem after scratching the root a little. This root is well-covered to protect the juice from outer dust. Juice coming out of the cut is gathered in vessels for 2 or 3 months. After that, when it is taken out-it appears like gum in final shape. This processed juice is 'Heeng', which is available in the market in two froms (i) golden brown round and flat pieces (ii) big pieces. Heera Heeng is supposed to be of the best quality.

Heeng is an expectorant, carminative, stimulant and powerful antispasmodic, antiseptic, germicidal, diuretic, laxative, antiphlegm.atic, anti-flatulent, stimulator of secretion and excretion, blood-purifier, pain-killer and tonic.

3. Chemical Properties of Heeng : –

Heeng has sulphyreted volatile oil 3 to 9%. This volatile oil chieflv consists of

Allyl Sulphide

Resin - 50-70% soluble in ether,

Gum - 30%.

Saline matters and ash - 3-4%.

It also has Ferualic, Malic, acetic, formic and valerianic acids.

4. Curative Properties of Heeng : –

Indigestion and stomach problems

(i) Taking 2 gms. of Hingasthak Churna (Grind Ajwain, black- pepper, Sendha Namak, Peepal, Kala Jeera, dry ginger and Heenga roasted in ghee and a little edible soda) after meals with lukewarm water cures all digestive problems.

(ii) Taking 1 tsp. of Hingashthak Churna with 1 tsp. of ground aniseed with water-cures uneasiness due to flatulence.

(iii) Taking lemon juice, ginger juice with little roasted Heeng powder and sendha namak in cold water-gives quick relief in flatulence.

(iv) Giving hot Heeng water (Heeng boiled in 250 gm. water till it is reduced to half) releases wind and gives relief in pain.

(v) Applying a solution of Heeng in hot water-near the navel region or taking roasted ground Heeng with any eatable activates appetite and eliminates digestive problems.

(vi) Taking one teaspoon of powder (made from grinding roasted Heeng, choti harar, sendha namak, Ajwain in equal quantity) 2 times a day cures indigestion.

(vii) Taking little Heeng mixed in water eliminates stomach uneasiness and wind.

Bite of Poisonous Insects : –

(i) Applying paste of ground Heeng with water eliminates poison.

(ii) Applying a little Heeng mixed with Ghee on the snake bitten part after pressing the poisoned blood to ooze out-is an antidote of poison.

(iii) Applying Heeng boiled in the Coconut milk (extracted from grated fresh coconut) on the scorpion bitten part-and keeping it wet for few minutes-will give relief.

Stomach-ache in children : —

(i) Applying a paste of roasted Heeng in ghee-cures taut stomach of the child.

(ii) Slightly rubbing Heeng dissolved in water on the upper stomach cures stomach-ache of the children.

Constipation : —

Taking Hingasthak Churn, Harar with sweet soda activates the movement of bowels.

Hiccoughs : —

Taking a pinch of Heeng with banana or Gur cures hiccoughs.

Headache : —

Applying solution of Heeng in water on the head relieves pain.

Pain in Ribs : —

Applying solution of Heeng (in water) on the ribs eliminates pain.

Tooth-ache : —

Keeping a pinch of Heeng on the tooth which is paining relieves pain and also destroys tooth-worms.

Foul breath : —

Taking Hingasthak Churna with food or with warm water cures all digestive problems and then clears the foul smell of breath.

Cold and Cough : —

(i) Smelling the solution of little Heeng with water-eliminates the deposited phlegm.

(ii) Taking Heeng roasted in ghee-forces down the trapped phlegm. which gets cleared by the bowel movement.

Hoarse Throat : —

(i) Gargling with hot water with little Heeng dissolved in it— restores normal voice.

(ii) Sucking a small piece of fresh ginger with Heeng powder sprinkled on it-releases all trapped phlegm. and makes the voice normal.

Bronchites : —

Taking water-with Munakka and little Heeng boiled in it- eliminates trouble caused by irritation of bronchial chords.

Pneumonia : —

(i) Taking little Heeng dissolved in water-gives quick relief in congestion.

(ii) Massaging the chest with oil (made by roasting ground Heeng and 4-5 cloves of garlic in oil) and covering it with some cloth-eliminates congestion.

Arthritis : —

(i) Massaging the affected part with oil (Boil Heeng, garlic and Sendha namak in equal proportion-in mustard oil. Strain it) and covering it with some cloth eliminates stiffness and pain.

(ii) Taking 1 cup of hot milk in which half a spoonful of this oil is added-before sleep-is also very helpful.

Hysteria : —

Smelling Heeng cures Hysteria.

Wounds : —

(i) Applying Heeng solution on the wound-eliminates pain and cures the wound easily.

(ii) Regular intake of Asafoetida Mother Tincture (Homeopathic medicine) cures all types of wounds.

Urticaria : —

Applying little Heeng fried in ghee on the affected part helps in curing it.

Low Blood Pressure : —

Taking roasted ground Heeng with water-boosts up blood pressure.

Weak Heart : —

(i) Taking roasted Heeng with water gives energy to heart, and purifies blood.

(ii) Taking little Churna (Grind finely 5 gms. of Heera Heeng, 12 munnakkas without seeds, 12 dried dates without stones, Dalchini and small cardamom–10 gms. each mixed with little sendha namak, strain and store it) taken 3-4 times a day strengthens the heart.

Obesity : —

Taking low calorie food with Heeng powder sprinkled on it- dissolves excess fat in the body.

Diarrhoea : —

Taking 1 tsp. Churna (Roast mango seed and take out its soft part and Roast Heeng also. Grind both with a little Sendha namak) stops loose motions.

Dysentery : —

Roast aniseed and Heeng separately in ghee and grind. Taking this powder with water-cures mucous and blood coming in stool.

Worms : —

(i) Giving pinch of Heeng to children is preventive against worms and helps in throwing out the dead worms if any.

(ii) Applying Heeng solution in water by cotton wool on rectum destroys worms (as sometimes they are seen coming from rectum.)

(iii) Giving enema of Heeng is very useful in throwing out worms.

Urinary problems : —

Taking little roasted Heeng dissolved in water cures burning sensation in urine.

Menstrual Disorders : —

Taking Heeng during menses cures menstrual disorders, increases menstrual flow and relieves of excessive pain during periods.

Anus-Itching in children : —

(i) Making the child drink solution of water with little Heeng-2 times a day-gives relief in itching.

(ii) Pouring Heeng-water with cotton wool externally-also gives immediate relief.

Delivery pains : —

Swallowing little Heeng (size of Bajra) kept in piece of Gur with one or two sips of water-helps in quick delivery.

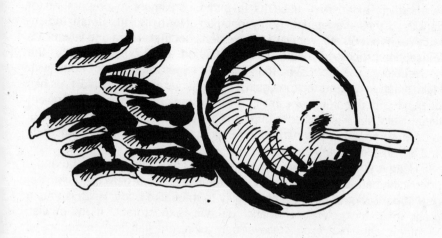

HALDI (Turmeric)

1. Haldi is known in different languges as : —

1.	Sanskrit	—	*Haridra, Kanchani, Pitta, Krmighna, Nisa, Yositapriya*
2.	Hindi	—	*Haldi*
3.	Latin	—	*Curcuma longa*
4.	Bengali	—	*Haridra, Halud*
5.	Marathi	—	*Halad*
6.	Kannada	—	*Arseena*
7.	Telegu	—	*Pasupu*
8.	Gujrati	—	*Haldar*
9.	Tamil	—	*Manjala,*
10.	Sindhi	—	*Haldi, Hedda,*
11.	English	—	*Turmeric*

2. Description : —

Haldi is grown and found all over India. Its plant is like ginger plant having 4-5 ft. height. Its leaves are pointed 6-7" wide and 1 to $1\frac{1}{2}$ ft. long and their smell is sweet, fragrant like the pollen of mango. The root has beautiful, captivating golden complexion, when taken out of ground. This is then dried in the sun and is known as Haldi.

Haldi is extensively used as favourite condiment in preparation of various dishes -vegetarian non-vegetarian, North Indian, South Indian, Mughlai, Tandoori etc., for without it we don't get that aroma and flavour. Its antiseptic properties helps in preservation of food. Not only the householders use it but even the seers and sages anoint their bodies with Haldi solution as a protection against the vagaries of nature. Haldi thus has been accorded a high place in all the rituals and ceremonies since ancient times. Haldi ubtan is applied to bride and bridegroom before marriage. Haldi is used commonly while performing Puja at religious and social functions and is considered very auspicious.

Haldi is stringent and sour in taste. It is a time-tested beauty aid and a nourishing herb-which not only gives natural gloss, royal glow and lustre but also imparts vigour and youthful vitality to the entire body. Haldi is thus a great tonic in general, aromatic, diuretic, expectorant, blood-purifier, skin-tonic, carminative, pain reliever, germicidal, anti-flatulent, producer and enhancer of red blood corpuscles, anti–phlegm.atic, antibilleous, protector of eyes, anti-inflammatory and imparts coolness to the system.

3. Chemical properties of Haldi :

Haldi contains volatile oil 1%, Resin, Curcumin, yellow-colouring matter, Turmeric oil or Turmer-oil. This turmeric oil is a thick oil, which is the cause of aromatic taste and smell of Haldi.

4. Curative Properties of Haldi : –

Bruises, sprain and wounds : –

(i) Applying past of Haldi powder with lime or water on the effected part-eliminates swelling and pain in bruises .

(ii) Taking 1 tsp. Haldi powder with hot milk is also useful.

(iii) Filling the wound or cut, (from which blood is coming out) with Haldi powder-will stop bleeding and curing of the wound/cut.

(iv) Applying poultice made of gram flour, Haldi powder mixed with mustard or Til oil-on the sprained portion-enhances blood circulation and gives relief.

(v) Tying a bandage of Haldi (prepared with 4 tsp. flour, 2 tsp. Haldi powder, 1 tsp. pure ghee, $\frac{1}{2}$ tsp. sendha Namak with water) on the bruised portion gives relief.

(vi) Giving fomentation with cloth soaked in hot water (500 gm. water boiled with $\frac{1}{2}$ tsp. Sendha Namak and 1 tsp. Haldi powder) on the bruised part eliminates pain and swelling.

(vii) Giving fomentation with Potli (having one ground onion mixed with 1 tsp. Haldi powder) heated with Til oil on the bruised portion gives relief.

(viii) Applying Haldi powder heated in Ghee or oil on the wound and tying it with a bandage helps in quick healing of the wound.

(ix) Dusting Haldi powder on wounds also helps.

Skin-problems :—

(i) Ringworm white spots :— applying paste of Haldi rubbed on stone with water on the effected portion is useful.

(ii) Skin eruptions :— Applying paste of Haldi and til oil on the body prevents skin eruptions.

(iii) Applying Haldi powder or paste on the body before bath is a preventive against skin problems and also a depilatory. (clears the growth of hair on body).

(iv) Urticaria : (a) Taking $\frac{1}{4}$ tsp. haldi powder with $\frac{1}{2}$ tsp. Mishri or honey twice a day cures urticaria.

(b) Taking Halwa (made from 2 tsp. flour, 1 tsp. ghee, $\frac{1}{2}$ tsp. haldi, 2 tsp. sugar, $\frac{1}{2}$ cup water) in the morning cures Utricaria.

(v) Taking roasted Haldi with Gur cures itching.

(vi) Eczema : sucking tablet of ground haldi with honey for 10-15 days cures Eczema.

(vii) Pustules : Placing cotton dipped in Haldi oil over pustules gives relief.

(viii) Freckles, spots : (a) Applying Haldi rubbed on stone with water eliminates them. (b) Massaging the face with Ubtan (mix ground Haldi with milk of banyan or pipal & soak it overnight) 1 hour before bath eliminates freckles on the face and imparts natural glow.

Cough & Cold, Asthma :—

(i) Taking Haldi powder and little salt with hot water or sucking a small piece of haldi or licking $\frac{1}{4}$ tsp. Haldi powder with 1 tsp. honey-gives relief in cough and eliminates congestion of bronchi.

(ii) Taking $\frac{1}{4}$ tsp. Haldi with hot milk is helpful in checking running nose.

(iii) Inhaling the smoke of burnt Haldi throws out the trapped phlegm.

(iv) Taking $\frac{1}{4}$ tsp. powder of Haldi (roasted in hot sand & then ground) with hot water relieves breathing problem (Asthma)

(v) Taking Haldi boiled in milk and sweetened with Jaggery is very useful in cold and Asthma.

(vi) Sucking a piece of Haldi (like lemon drops) or keeping it in mouth at night cures chronic cold.

(vii) Licking tablets (made by mixing Haldi powder, barley powder and bansa-ash in equal proportion and honey and making small tablets) 4-5 times in a day eliminates trapped phlegm. in the body.

(viii) Massaging the throat & chest with little Haldi powder, ground black pepper mixed with ghee-cures irritation in bronchial chords.

(ix) Giving a pinch of Haldi powder with milk to children gives quick relief.

(x) Inhaling smoke of cow-dung cake with Haldi sprinkled on it- releases the trapped phlegm.

(xi) Taking $\frac{1}{4}$ tsp. of Haldi powder with 3-4 gulps of warm water-acts as a preventive against attack of Asthma.

Whooping cough : —

(i) Taking $\frac{1}{4}$ tsp. ground roasted Haldi powder with two spoons of honey 3 or 4 times a day gives relief in cough.

(ii) Taking Pan with little Haldi piece in it is also useful.

Indigestion & stomach problems : —

(i) Taking Haldi powder and salt in equal quantity with warm water gives instant relief in acidity.

(ii) Taking 1 tsp. Churna (Grind Haldi 4 gm., Sonth 4 gm., Black pepper 2 gm. and Ilayachi 2 gm.) after meals is digestive, eliminates wind and stomach ailments.

(iii) Taking curd or whey with Haldi powder after lunch cures digestive problems.

Leech-bite : —

Applying paste of Haldi powder stops bleeding from leech-bite.

Sore-Throat : —

Licking Haldi powder mixed with honey 2-3 times a day cures soreness.

Tonsilitis : —

Fomentation with paste made of 10 gm. Haldi powder roasted in mustard oil and then tied around the neck gives relief in Tonsils.

Blisters in mouth : —

Gargling with 1 glass water in which little Haldi powder is boiled, twice a day, cures it.

Urinary Troubles : —

• Taking paste of ground or juice of raw Haldi and honey with goat's milk (if available) twice a day, cures all urinary problems.

Small-pox : —

(i) Taking $\frac{1}{4}$ tsp. powder of Haldi and Imli (tamarind) for 4-5 days acts as a preventive against small-pox.

(ii) Applying a thin layer of the ubtan (Haldi powder, foam of fresh milk and Wheat flour mixed with mustard oil or fresh cream) on the affected part twice a day-flattens the deep spots of Small-pox and makes the skin soft.

Worms : –

Licking the paste (made of $\frac{1}{4}$ tsp. Haldi powder and $\frac{1}{2}$ tsp. Vayavidang Choorna with 1 tsp. of honey-for 7-8 days kills worms and throws them out.

Pregnancy and postnatal care : –

(i) Taking 5-10 gms. of Haldi powder with water-during menses is an antipregnancy dose for ladies.

(ii) Taking $\frac{1}{4}$ tsp. with hot milk in latter part of the 9th month of pregnancy helps in easy delivery.

(iii) Taking $\frac{1}{2}$ tsp. roasted Haldi powder with Gur after delivery eliminates weakness and cures uterus swelling.

Pain in breasts : –

Applying paste of Haldi rubbed on stone on the affected part eliminates pain.

Gout : –

Taking Laddu of Haldi (mix $\frac{1}{2}$ kg. roasted ground Haldi, one finely grated dried Coconut 1 kg. jaggery, 200 gm. cashew nuts or ground nuts and make laddu) daily in the morning with Tulsi or lemon tea-makes the joints supple and gives relief in pain and swelling.

Pain in Ribs : –

(i) Applying paste of Haldi powder mixed in hot water-on the aching ribs gives relief or

(ii) Massaging the ribs with Haldi oil or

(iii) Massaging the ribs with paste of Haldi powder in milk of the Aak plant gives quick relief.

Jaundice & Liver problems : –

Taking 4-5 gms. of Haldi powder mixed in a glass of whey twice a day activates the liver.

Diabetes : –

Taking 4-5 gms. ground Haldi with water or honey twice a day is helpful in curing diabetes.

Leucorrhoea : –

(i) Taking Haldi powder with sugar twice a day for sometime checks this.

(ii) Washing the private parts with Haldi water (10 gm. Haldi boiled in 100 gm. water) is also useful. Alongwith it taking one Batasha with 8-10 drops of milk of Banyan tree before sunrise for 7 days helps in early cure.

Debility in Males :–

Taking about 7-8 gms. of raw ground Haldi and equal amount of honey with goat's milk (preferably) cures debility in males.

Dental Problems :–

(i) Rinsing the mouth with Haldi water (Boil 5 gms. Haldi powder, 2 clove and 2 dried leaves of Guava in 200 gms. water) gives instant relief.

(ii) Applying and rubbing the teeth with paste of Haldi powder, salt and mustard oil-strengthens the gums.

(iii) Massaging the aching teeth with roasted ground Haldi eliminates pain and swelling.

(iv) Keeping piece of roasted Haldi near the aching tooth and letting the saliva ooze out also helps.

(v) Filling the cavity in teeth-with roasted ground Haldi powder -gives relief from pain.

(vi) Applying the powder of burnt Haldi piece and Ajwain on teeth and cleaning them makes the gums and teeth strong.

Ear troubles :–

Putting one or two drops of Haldi (by roasting 2 pieces of Haldi in mustard oil) in the ear, cleaning it with an ear-bud cures ear-problems.

Eye-troubles :–

(i) Cloth dipped in the solution of Haldi powder and water is employed as an eye-shade.

(ii) Dropping Haldi water ($\frac{1}{4}$ tsp. Haldi powder boiled in 500 gms. water till 125 gm. water is left. Cool and strain it through a fine cloth) in the eyes twice a day and putting the cotton soaked in water on the eyelids relieves pain, redness, irritation and itching in the eyes.

(iii) Applying bit heated paste of piece of Haldi rubbed on stone on eyelids also eliminates pain, swelling and eye-troubles.

(iv) A decoction of Haldi powder with water as a cooling lotion on the eyes is useful in conjunctivities.

Poison of Insect-bite :–

Applying the mixture of Haldi powder and lime over the affected part nullifies the toxic effect.

Coryza :–

Inhalations of fumes of burning Haldi passed into the nostrils relieves coryza.

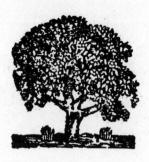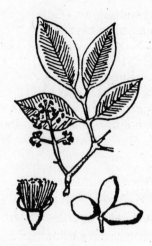

JAMUN (Jambul Tree)

1. Jamun is known in different languages as : —

1.	Sanskrit	—	*Mahajambu, Mahaphala, Nandis, Phalendra*
2.	Hindi	—	*Jamun*
3.	Latin	—	*Eugenia Jambolana*
4.	Bengali	—	*Kalajam*
5.	Marathi	—	*Nadi Jambhula*
6.	Kannada	—	*Dohuniratu*
7.	Telegu	—	*Peddaneradi*
8.	Gujrati	—	*Jambuna*
9.	Tamil	—	*Shambu*
10.	Sindhi	—	*Jammu*
11.	English	—	*Jambul tree*

2. Description : —

Jamun tree is found all over India. It is sufficiently high and remains green throughout the year. Its leaves are 2-3" wide and 3-6" long. Bunch of small white flowers with green tinge appears from March to May and the dark mauve-coloured fruits ripen during rainy season. There are two varieties :

(1) Rajajambu - Grown by grafting. Its fruit is very tasty and is large in size with lots of pulp and small seed.

69

(2) Kathajamun - Grown by seeds. Its fruit is little sour, small in size with less pulp and a big seed.

Its bark and seed is used for preparing medicines. Its bark is used for leather dyeing and tanning. Its wood is very strong and durable and boats are made from it.

Jamun fruit is sweet and tasty. It helps in digestion, acts as an appetiser and diuretic, particularly useful in diabetes, controls cough and bile.

Jamun trees are found in abundance in Bhagalpur (Bihar) and Bankuda, Purulia (Bengal) where silk-worms for making Tassar-silk are reared on the tree.

Precaution : –

Milk should never be taken immediately after eating Jamun.

3. Chemical Properties of Jamun : –

It contains the following :

Glucocide (Jambolin), Elegic Acid, Yellow Fragrant Oil, Fat, Raal, Gelic Acid, Albumin.

Its bark contains 12% Tannin.

3. Curative Properties of Jamun : –

Diabetes : –

(i) 3-5 gms. of powdered seed with or without salt 2 times a day taken for some time eliminates sugar.

(ii) 2 tsp. powder of dry fruit of Jamun taken 2 times a day or

(iii) Intake of fresh Jamun fruit is recommended.

Excessive Bleeding : –

$\frac{1}{2}$ tsp. to 1 tsp. powdered bark of Jamun tree taken with milk stops excessive bleeding.

Diaherrhoea : – .

Powdered Guthali (seed) taken with $\frac{1}{2}$ cup water taken 2-3 times cures-loose motions and blood.

Strangury : –

Jamun juice or sharbat taken 2-3 times a day for somedays cures strangury.

Urinating while asleep : –

One tsp. of powdered Guthali (seed) of Jamun taken with fresh water especially at night checks the habit of urinating in bed while asleep.

Night Discharge : –

4 gm. powdered Jamun Guthli (seed) taken with water morning and evening cures night discharge.

Vomiting : –

Taking boiled juice of Jamun & mango leaves (in equal quantity) cures Vomiting.

Leucarrhoea : –

Powder of innerseed of Guthali of Jamun taken with biled rice water for some time-cures leucrrhoea.

Stomach Problems : –

(i) 4-8 gm. of Vinegar made of Jamun juice twice a day with little salt cures stomach-ache, indigestion, loss of appetite, problem of spleen and liver.

(ii) Jamun juice with a little sendha Namak cures stomach- problems

Stone : –

Taking fresh Jamun fruit or powdered Guthali of Jamun with curd eliminates stone.

Wounds : –

Paste of Jamun leaves applied on wounds heals them.

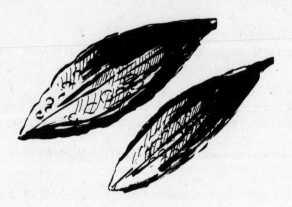

KARELA (Hairy Mordica)

1. Karela is known in different languages as : —

1.	Sanskrit	—	*Karavella, Kathilla*
2.	Hindi	—	*Karela, Kareli*
3.	Latin	—	*Memordica Charantia*
4.	Bengali	—	*Bada Karela Uchhe, Chot Karela Uchh*
5.	Marathi	—	*Karlen, Kshudra Karali*
6.	Kannada	—	*Hagalakai*
7.	Telegu	—	*Karila, Kakarkaya*
8.	Gujrati	—	*Karelun*
9.	Sindhi	—	*Karela*
10.	English	—	*Hairy Mordica*

2. Description : —

Karela is very bitter in taste. It is a rich source of Phosphorous. The needs of Phosphorous in human body are fulfilled by taking one Karela a day. Regular use of Karela is invigorating and keeps one active.

Karela is a blood purifier, activates spleen and liver and is highly beneficial in Diabetes. It is a purgative, appetiser, digestive, anti-inflammatory, antiflatulent and has healing capacity.

72

3. Composition :—

Wala	-	92.4 %
Minerals	-	0.8 %
Protein	-	1.6 %
Fat	-	4.2
Carbohydrates	-	4.2
Calcium	-	0.03
Phosphorous	-	0.07

100 gms. of Karela contain

22 mg	-	Iron
210 (International Unit)	-	Vitamin A
24 "	-	Vitamin B
88 mg	-	Vitamin C

4. Curative Properties of Karela :—

Arthrites :—

Massage the affected portion with juice of Karela and eat Karela vegetable to cure pain in joints.

Diabetes :—

(i) Juice of Karela 5-10 gms. with or without water taken 3 times a day for 2-3 months-eliminates sugar problem. or (ii) 3-6 gms. ground Karela (cut into pieces, dried in shade and then ground) fresh water taken for 2 to 3 months is useful. In addition to the above-vegetable of Karela is also recommended.

Leucorrhoea :—

$\frac{1}{2}$ tsp. of Karela juice 2 times a day- taken for some time cures leucorrhoea.

Jaundice :—

1-2 tsp. of ground fresh juice of Karela with water-twice a day cures jaundice. (Note - Adminstration of juice should be stopped when the yellow appearance in eyes ceases).

Liver :—

$\frac{1}{2}$ tsp. of Karela juice given to child of 3-8 yrs. daily is a preventive against liver problems. In enlarged liver-50 gm. juice with water is advised.

(ii) Taking juice of Karela (after boiling it) or fresh juice helps in curing liver troubles.

Worms :—

1 tsp. Karela juice daily for sometime destroys worms.

Piles :—

1 tsp. Karela juice with sugar - 2 times a day, stops oozing of blood from piles.

Constipation :—

(i) Taking 5-10 drops of homeopathic medicine 'Momradica Charantia' (made from Karela) - 4 times a day cures constipation.

(ii) $\frac{1}{2}$ tsp. juice of Karela twice a day is digestive.

Blood Purifier :—

1-2 tsp. of Karela juice in the morning taken for few days purifies blood.

Precaution : —

(i) Karela generates heat and is harmful if taken in exessive quantity.

(ii) Curd or lemon are useful in case of disorder caused by its excessive use.

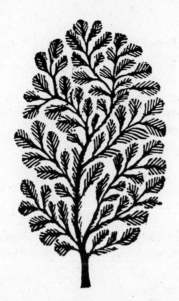

JEERA (Cumin Seeds)

1. Jeera is known in different languages as :—

1.	Sanskrit	—	*Jiraka, Jarana, Ajajikana, Dirgha-Jiraka*
2.	Hindi	—	*Jeera Safed*
3.	Latin	—	*Cuminum Cyminum*
4.	Bengali	—	*Jeere*
5.	Marathi	—	*Jeeren*
6.	Kannada	—	*Jeerige*
7.	Telegu	—	*Jeekri, Jeelakari*
8.	Gujrati	—	*Jeerum*
9.	Tamil	—	*Jeerakam*
10.	Sindhi	—	*Jeero*
11.	English	—	*Cuminseeds*

2. Description :—

Jeera, especially beneficial in Indian climate, is one of the most common condiments used in preparing vegetables, Dals, pickles and any vegetarian and non-vegetarian dishes. Jeera is extensively used for preparing various medicines in Unani and Ayurvedic systems.

It is usually grown all over India. Its plant is $1\frac{1}{2}$ ft to 3 ft high and leaves are very small. Its fruit is small in size but long in shape. It has three varieties (1) Safed Jeera (ii) Kala Jeera (iii) Kalongie and all the varieties are used.

Jeera is dry, a bit astringent, carminative, stomachic, aromatic, blood-purifier. It is stimulant used in dyspepsia, diarrhoea, fever, swelling, uterus problems and is germicidal insecticide.

3. Chemical Properties of Jeera : —

Jeera (cumin seeds) have Fat Oil	7.7 p.c
Resin	13.5 p.c
Gum and Mucilage	8.00 p.c
Proteins	15.5 p.c

It contains essential oil which has its special aromatic odour on which its taste depends. This oil has : — Cuminal 56% a mixture of hydro-carbons, cymene or cymol terpene.

4. Curative Properties of Jeera : —

Mouth Ailments : —

(i) Eating roasted Jeera eliminates foul smell in the mouth.

(ii) Gargling with ground Jeera put in water with crushed choti ilyachi eliminates foul smell and cures blisters in the mouth.

(iii) Applying powder of ground roasted Jeera and sendha Namak (in equal quantity) on the gums-and then leaving the saliva to ooz out helps in reducing the swelling of gums and cures the pain.

Indigestion and stomach problems : —

(i) Taking Jeera water (1 tsp. Jeera boiled in 1 glass of water cool and strain it. Make 3 doses of it)-thrice a day eliminates indigestion.

(ii) Taking 1 tsp. of churna (Grind Jeera, sonth, sendha namak, pippali, black pepper in equal quantity. Store it in a bottle) with water after meals is a digestive which stimulates hunger. It eliminates wind and gas.

(iii) Taking ground Jeera with honey or jaggery after meals cures stomache-ache.

Diarrhoea : —

(i) Taking roasted ground jeera powder mixed with $\frac{1}{2}$ tsp. honey controls loose motions.

(ii) Taking roasted ground jeera in whey after meals checks diarrhoea.

Stranguary : —

Taking ground Jeera with honey helps in controlling urine problems.

Leucorrhoea : —

Taking ground roasted Jeera with sugar controls leucorrhoea.

Post-Delivery problems : –

(i) Taking water in which Jeera powder is mixed-acts as an antiseptic and helps in shrinking of ovaries to their normal size.

(ii) Taking this Jeera water is useful in other problems of menses after delivery.

(iii) Eating vegetables with Jeera fried in Ghee increases the milk in the breasts.

(iv) Taking 10 gms. of roasted Jeera and sugar with 100 gms. milk aslo increases the milk in the breasts.

(v) Taking chapatis made of dough in which Jeera and Ajwain have been kneaded-helps the mother get enough milk in her breasts.

(vi) Taking decoction made of Jeera given just after delivery- stimulates the uterus to contract to its original position.

(vii) Taking Jeera with Gur is very beneficial for uterus- contraction.

Piles : –

(i) Taking Jeera with Mishri helps in curing piles.

(ii) Taking 1 cup water (Boil-Jeera, sonf, Cordiander seeds-1 tsp. each in a glass of water till one cup is left) with pure ghee eliminates oozing of blood in piles.

(iii) Taking 1 tsp. ground Jeera and $\frac{1}{4}$ tsp. ground black pepper with honey eliminates pain and cures piles.

Urticaria : –

Taking bath with water having Jeera boiled in it – cures urticaria and itching.

Spots, freckles : –

(i) Applying paste (made from ground Jeera, Kala Til, and sarson in equal quantity mixed in milk) on face eliminates spots and freckles and imparts a natural softness and glow.

(ii) Washing the face with water in which Jeera is boiled beautifies the skin.

Chronic Fever : –

(i) Taking Jeera with Gur twice a day for 3 weaks cures chronic fever.

(ii) Taking 3-4 gms. of churna of Jeera (Boil Jeera in Cow's milk-when dried-grind it) with Mishri regularly cures chronic fever.

Swelling of hands and feet : –

Applying paste of Jeera powder with water removes painful swellings of hands and feet.

Hoarse throat : –

Gargles with Jeera water eliminates hoarseness of throat.

Insect-bite :—

(i) Applying a paste of Jeera and sonth on the affected part (in case of spider) eliminates the poison.

(ii) Taking ground Jeera and black pepper in water (in case of dog-bite) eliminates poison.

(iii) Applying heated paste of ground Jeera with Sendha Namak and ghee in case of scorpion bite eliminates poison.

Worms :—

Taking 1 tsp. Jeera with water before going to bed for 2 or 3 days kills the worms.

Insect-repellant :—

(i) Keeping a little bundle of Jeera in cup boards-makes them free from insects.

(ii) Keeping Jeera seeds between woollen shawls and clothes acts as a protection against insects.

General Tonic :—

(i) Taking 2-3 gms. of ground Jeera boiled in 100 gms. of water for 5 minutes with milk and sugar to taste-gives energy and vigour to the whole body.

(ii) Eating Kheer of 20 gms. Jeera (soak Jeera in 250 gms. milk for 2 hours. Cook on slow fire till it gets thickened. Mix sugar or Mishri to your taste) stimulates digestion and stengthens physicals and mental faculties.

Precaution :—

Pregnant ladies should not take Jeera in exchessive quantity for it may lead to 'ABORTION'.

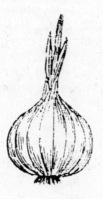

LAHSUN (Garlic)

1. Lahsun is known in different languages as :—

1.	Sanskrit	—	*Lashuna, Rasona*
2.	Hindi	—	*Lahsun*
3.	Latin	—	*Allium Sativum*
4.	Bengali	—	*Rashun*
5.	Marathi		*Lasuna*
6.	Kannada		*Bellulli*
7.	Telegu	—	*Tellbulli*
8.	Gujrati	—	*Lasana*
9.	Tamil	—	*Vallaipandu*
10.	Sindhi	—	*Thumma*
11.	English	—	*Garlic Root*

2. Description :—

According to Pauranic legends, Lahsun originated from drop of nectar dropped from sky in a scuffle between Indra & Garuda and so it is called 'Amritodbhava'. It is also called 'Rason', because it contains all 'Rasas' except Amlarasa'. This be speaks of its high therapeutic value.

Lahsun plant is a delicate plant 1-2 ft in height, with long, cylindrical leaves, which surround the stem bearing white flowers (in-florscense). The root, which is underground has many parts each of the shape of barley &

that is the 'edible part'. This is of 2 types (i) Rason &(ii) Maharason & is grown all over India.

Lahsun is a gastric stimulant & helps in digestion, acts as an anti-flatulant, carminative and diaphoretic. It is stimulant of Kidneys and skin and is diuretic in nature. It is a tonic giving strength & vitality, an expectorant having a special effect on the bronchial and Pulmonary secretions, beneficial for eyes and brain and helps in healing fractured bones and is a great antiseptic. It has "Allicin"-which has the property to destroy even those germs-which are not killed by Pennincillin. It is thus a very powerful germicidal.

3. Chemical Composition of Lahsun : —

It has volatile oil, starch, mucilage 35%, albumen, etc.

Carbohydrates	29.00%,	Protein	6.3%
Fat	0.1 ,,	Mineral salts	1.0 ,,
Volatile Oil	0.06 ,,	Phosphorus	0.31 ,,
Lime	0.03,,		

Apart from this 100 gm of Lahsun contains Iron – 1.3 gm, sufficient quantity of Vitamin A, B, C, sugar minerals like Albumen, Mangnese, Chlorine, lead and copper.

Oil of Garlic is Volatile Oil – obtained by distillation. It contains allyl, propyl, disulphide, diallyl disulphide and other sulpher compounds. Its colour is dark brown or yellow, taste- repungent & odour repulsive & has medical properties.

Curative and therapeutic Properties of Lahsun : —

Asthma : —

(i) Lahsun juice taken with hot water twice a day.

(ii) One fried shellot (Kali of Lahsun) with little salt – twice a day.

(iii) 10 drops of Lahsun juice with 2 teaspoon of honey-cures Asthma. It can be administered at the time of attack also.

Tuberclosis (T.B.) : —

Pulmonary infections including T.B. is controlled by :

(i) Regular in take of Lahsun – because its rich contents of Sulphuric Acid, destroys T.B. germs.

(ii) Chewing 10 shellots of Lahsun boiled in 250 gm. milk & then having that milk helps in curing T.B.

(iii) Chewing of 3-4 shellots of Lahsun 3 times a day reduces cough, increases appetite, induces sleep and helps in curing T.B. of lungs.

(iv) Smelling cotton-wool soaked in Lahsun juice carries its strong foul smell to Lungs which helps' in destroying all germs.

Heart Problems : —

(i) As diluting agent for blood — regular eating of Lahsun & then having milk with Lahsun boiled in it controls assimilation of cholestrol.

(ii) Chewing 4 or 5 shellots of Lahsun — given at the time of heart-attack — prevents heart failure and advised till medical aid is procured.

Paralysis : —

(i) 25 gms. ground Lahsun shellots boiled in milk — till it becomes thick (like Kheer) — to be taken when cooled in the morning for atleast a month.

Also massage the body with oil. (Boil 250 gms ground Lahsun shellots with 500 gm mustard oil in an iron Karahi (pan) till it is burnt. Put some camphor in it. Cool it & keep it in bottle for massage).

(ii) Eating 7 ground shellots of Lahsun with one tsp of fresh butter also helps in curing paralysis.

High Blood pressure : —

Taking 6 drops of lahsun juice with fresh water regularly reduces hypertension.

Bronchitis : —

Paste of garlic with onion applied on the chest as poultice cures bronchitis.

Bile, Cough, Wind : —

For bile — use of ground garlic with sugar; for cough with honey (especially in winter & spring) & for wind — with ghee (especially in rainy season) is highly recommended.

Whooping Cough, Cold & Cough : —

(i) Regular intake of 3-5 shallots of Lahsun cures cold & cough.

(ii) 6-7 drops of Lahsun juice mixed with Sharbat of Pomegranate cures all types of cold & cough — & even whooping cough.

(iii) Taking 1 shellot of Lahsun with 5 soaked, peeled & ground almonds and Mishri in the morning taken for 3-4 days cures whooping cough.

(iv) 8-10 drops of Lahsun juice mixed with 4 gms of honey — 4 times a day — cures whooping cough.

(v) Making the child wear a mala (garland) having 2 shellots of Lahsun — helps in curing whooping cough.

(vi) 5 drops of Lahsun in hot water given 2 or 3 times a day cures frequent and violent coughing spells.

Sore Throat : —

Gargles with hot water with few drops of Lahsun cures sore throat.

Sneezing : –

Juice of 5 to 7 shellots of Lahsun with hot water taken once stops frequent sneezing.

Malaria : –

Application of Lahsun juice on nails of hands and feet before fever & taking 1 tsp Lahsun juice with 1 tsp fresh water thrice a day cures malaria.

Jaundice : –

4 ground shellots of Lahsun mixed with half cup hot milk for 4-5 days helps in curing jaundice.

Impotency : –

Keep 200 gms ground Lahsun mixed with 600 gm. pure honey in a bottle – in a sack of wheat for 21 or 31 days.

(i) Taking 10 gms of that paste – followed by drinking lukewarm milk early in the morning for 21 or 31 days – gives exra- ordinary strength and helps in curing impotency.

(ii) Chewing 4 shellots of Lahsun slowly early in the morning – followed by drinking luke-warm milk or taking ghee – regularly in winters gives extra-ordinary strength to men. It removes infertility in women.

Night-discharge : –

Chewing 1-2 shellot of Lahsun with 1 cup hot milk before bedtime stops night-discharge.

Migraine : –

Paste of Lahsun applied on forehead or near the ears for 3-4 minutes and putting 2 drops of Lahsun juice in the nostril (of the affected side) relieves pain of migraine.

Ear-ache : –

Drop of Lahsun juice boiled in little mustard oil relieves ear-ache.

Pain in arms, legs : –

Fried ground Lahsun and Sonth in ghee mixed with honey be kept in bottle. Taking 10 gms of this & drinking hot milk, tea or coffee in winters relieves pain.

Arthrites : –

(i) Massage the body with Lahsun oil (250 gms. ground Lahsun shellots boiled in 500 gm mustard oil till Lahsun in burnt in an iron Karahi)

(ii) Take pieces of 3 or 4 shellots of Lahsun boiled in milk or kheer made of ground 3 or 4 shellots in milk before going to bed.

This has to be taken regularly with gradual increase in quantity for 6 weeks or more to cure arthirites.

Gastric ulcer & Acidity : –

After 2 or 3 sips of water taking ground shellot Lahsun (like pea in quantity) after meals – & drinking little water cures gastric ulcer, hypertension & other ailments due to atmospheric and water-pollution. As a stomachic –

eating Lahsun shellots – checkes excesive stomach acidity.

Diarrhoea : –

Taking 2 or 3 shellots of Lahsun with water has a soothing effect on varied types of diarrhoea.

Flatulence, Sciatica : –

Small dose of decoction (strain after boiling together 6 ounces of Lahsun with 2 pints of water and 4 pints of milk till the water is evaporated) given regularly cures flatulence, sciatica.

Round-worms : –

Intake of 1 Lahsun shellot for sometime acts as a vermifuge in expelling round-worms.

Frost-bite, Leucoderma, Ringworm, Alopecia : –

Apart from eating raw Lahsun – local application of Lahsun paste on affected part for 2 to 4 minutes is advisable.

Itching : –

Massaging the body with Lahsun oil purifies blood & cures itching.

Urinary problems : –

Paste of Lahsun applied below navel relieves strangury.

Infantile Convulsions : –

Poultice of Lahsun applied to the spine is recommended.

Polio : –

Regular Chewing 4-5 shellots of Lahsun – early in the morning cures polio.

Pyorrhoea : –

(i) Regularly taking 6-10 drops of Lahsun in 1 tsp. of honey cures pyorrhoea.

(ii) Boil Lahsun in mustard oil. When Lahsun gets fried – strain the oil, cool it & mix it with fried ground 30 gm. Ajwayan & 15 gm. Sendha salt.

Brushing the teeth with this cures bad breath and pyorrhoea. It is to be done for 2-3 months.

Baldness : –

Applying Lahsun juice on the bald head & leaving it to dry – 3 times a day for few weeks – helps in hair-growth.

Bites of Venomous Reptiles, dogs & other noxions strongs :−

(i) Paste of Lahsun applied on the bites of Venomous reptiles Counteracts poison.

(ii) 5-7 ground shellots of Lahsun mixed with $\frac{1}{2}$ pint of milk − adminstered immediately after bite − Counteracts the poison.

Hysteria :−

In haling the smell of shellots of Lahsun kept near the nostrils helps to recover from swooning.

Antiseptic for cleaning Wounds :−

Mixture of Lahsun juice & water is very effective antiseptic lotion for cleaning all types of wounds etc.

Lahsun is scientifically admitted & proved to be very useful and good for health. It can be classified as a therapeutic food − used raw or in cooking. Because of its medicinal and curative properties, it is a panacea for a number of ailments. It is rightly called 'king of Herbs' easily available to rich and poor alike.

Some people, however, disapprove of Lahsun because of its disagrreable strong odour. To prevent or suppress odour of Lahsun the following may be noted :−

(i) Chewing roasted coffee grains or fresh parsley leaves or cardamom seeds or fresh coriander leaves or washing out the mouth with lemon juice or eating apples − diminishes the odour of Lahsun.

(ii) Lemon juice or Vinegar put in LAHSUN − suppresses its odour.

Smell of Lahsun from hands can be removed by sprinkling the hands with salt and cleaning them properly with cold water.

Precautions :−

(i) In large doses it is an irritant and produces flatulence, headache, nausea, vomitting etc. So it should be taken in limited quantity.

(ii) As a local stimulant and irritant, it reddens the skin and causes Vesication. So its application should not be for more than 2-3 minutes.

(iii) Not Admissible for pregnant woman.

LAUNG (Cloves)

1. Laung is known in different languages as : —

1.	Sanskrit	—	*Lavanga, Deva-Kusuma, Sri-sangya*
2.	Hindi	—	*Lavanga, Laung*
3.	Latin	—	*Caryophyllus Aromaticus*
4.	Bengali	—	*Lavanga*
5.	Marathi	—	*Lavang*
6.	Kannada	—	*Lavang-kalika*
7.	Telegu	—	*Lavangalu, Karavallu*
8.	Gujrati	—	*Lavinga*
9.	Tamil	—	*Kiramver, Kirambu*
10.	Sindhi	—	*Laung*
11.	English	—	*Clove*

2. Description : —

Clove is grown in abundance in Penang, Ceylon, Jawa, Janjibar its near by islands and southern parts of India. Its tree 40-50 ft high retains its greenery even during autumn and has intoxicating fragrance in it.

Clove is calyx-tube of the flowers of the tree. These calyx-tubes are red in colour when plucked. Then they are spread for 2-3 days on big mats for drying. These cloves are bitter and aromatic in taste.

Clove is cool, stimulant of skin, kidney, liver, bronchi and increases circulation and raises blood-heat. It is aromatic, general stomachic, anti-emetic, local anaesthetic and antiseptic. It is carminative, anti-gastric, anti-flatulent, anti-phlegmatic, pain killer and anti-pyreutic.

3. Chemical Properties of clove : –

Clove contains heavy volatile oil-18%; Caryophyllin-a camphor, resin 6%. It also has caryophllic Acid, crystalline body, tannin, woody fibre, gum etc.

4. Curative properties of Laung : –

(i) Taking 2 or 3 drops of Clove Oil in sugar cures indigestion, intestinal problems and also diarrhoea.

(ii) Taking Cloves as flavouring agent-corrects griping caused by purgative and relieves flatulence.

(iii) Taking clove in combination with other spices and sendha Namak relieves indigestion, vomiting and quenches thirst.

(iv) Taking two ground clove put in warm water eliminates nausea, gas and indigestion.

(v) Chewing clove is also useful in nausea.

(vi) Chewing 1 clove twice after meals or taking it in Sharbat cures all acidic problems.

(vii) Taking clove in Paan or 1/4 tsp ground Clove, little rock salt with lukewarm water after meals relieves flatulence.

(viii) Taking a Clove lightly roasted in ghee, after meals releases all trapped wind in the body.

(ix) Taking 1 gm Clove churna (made by grinding clove, sonth, Ajwain and sendha Namak 3 gms each) twice a day cures all digestive problems and increases appetite.

Weakness after illness : –

Taking clove boiled water (water in which the cloves have been boiled) imparts resistance to fight against infections and ailments.

Cough, Throat problems : –

(i) Sucking the juice of roasted clove-cures itching in the throat.

(ii) Keeping Clove in mouth releases trapped phlegm and eliminates foul smell of the mouth.

(iii) Taking little powder of clove and Anar rind (in equal quantity) mixed with honey 2-3 times a day cures coughing.

(iv) Sucking 2 cloves roasted on Tawa eliminates phlegm.

Whooping Cough : –

Taking roasted ground clove with honey gives relief.

Hoarseness of Throat : –

(i) Chewing Clove and sucking its juice soothens vocal chords.

(ii) Chewing Clove with Mishri is also beneficial.

(iii) Keeping the clove (roasted on the flame of a candle) in mouth eliminates foul smell of breath and cures sore-throat.

Headache : –

(i) Applying paste of clove or clove-oil curves headache.

(ii) Taking 2-3 clove water (cloves boiled in 1 cup water till half is left) twice a day cures headache.

Hiccoughs : –

Taking water of 1-2 cloves (cloves soaked in lukewarm water) relieves hiccoughs.

Influenza : –

Taking 1/4 tsp powdered cloves and pipali, 1/4 tsp ginger juice with 1 tsp honey 3-4 times a day gives relief.

Pneumonia : –

Taking Paan leaf with a little clove oil spread on it and Mishjri-early in the morning and Paan with a clove after meals clears congestion and brings relief.

Fever : –

Taking powder of 1 clove with warm water 3 times a day checks fever.

Malaria : –

(i) Taking one clove heated in pure ghee and Tulsi leaf-early in morning is preventive against Malaria.

(ii) Taking tea with clove and Tulsi leaves boiled in it eliminates malaria.

Typhoid : –

Taking clove water (Boil 5 cloves in 2kg water till 1kg is left. Strain and cool it) is useful in Typhoid.

Asthma : –

Taking 3-4 roasted cloves before going to bed-eliminates congestion in the chest and gives relief in breathing.

Measles : –

Taking one clove rubbed with water on stone with honey gives relief.

Worms : –

(i) Taking clove water whenever thirsty throws out worms.

(ii) Chewing one clove after dinner before eating a ripe small roasted tomato-also helps in throwing out worms.

Stranguary : –

Taking clove with water 2-3 times a day helps in curing this.

Ulcer : —

Applying paste of cloves and Haldi cures ulcer.

Bite of poisonous Insects : —

Applying paste of clove (rubbed with water on stone) on affected part gives relief.

Rheumatic-pain : —

Applying paste of clove on affected part gives relief.

Excessive thirst : —

Drinking boiling hot water of clove-quenches excessive thirst.

Teeth care and problems : —

(i) Rubbing the teeth with ground clove and lemon juice cures tooth-ache and makes the teeth shining.

(ii) Gargling with clove water (3-4 cloves boiled in 1 glass water) 2-3 times a day-cures tooth ache.

(iii) Pressing cotton soaked in clove oil on the cavity in tooth-eliminates pain.

(iv) Applying clove-oil on affected teeth before going to bed-for some days checks foul smell and cures Pyrrhoea.

(v) Taking roasted clove-strengthens gums and teeth.

Stye : —

Applying clove rubbed on stone with water-on the stye eliminates swelling and helps in curing stye.

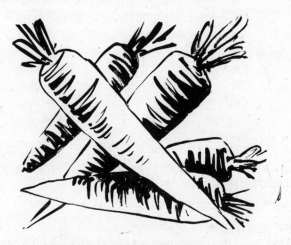

MULI (Radish)

1. Muli is known in different languages as : —

1.	Sanskrit	—	*Mulaka, Hasthidantaka*
2.	Hindi	—	*Muli*
3.	Latin	—	*Raphanus Sativus*
4.	Bengali	—	*Mula*
5.	Marathi	—	*Mula*
6.	Telegu	—	*Mulegi*
7.	Gujrati	—	*Mula*
8.	Tamil	—	*Mulegi*
9.	Sindhi	—	*Muree*
10.	English	—	*Radish.*

2. Description : —

Radish is a available all over India and almost throughout the year. Its plant is 1ft to $1\frac{1}{2}$ft in height. Its root, which is white or pink in colour, lies under ground. According to Ayurveda Radish is unparalleled in curing stomach ailments. The seeds, stalks, bean, root, leaves of radish-are all edibles. It is a unique root having hot and cold affect on the body simultaneously. It is acidic in reaction and pungent in smell.

Radish is digestive, antistomachaic, diuretic, blood-purifier, lessens nervous tensions and helps in enhancing blood circulation. It is germicidal and suppresses wind, bile and phlegm.

3. Chemical Properties of Radish : —

100 gms of radish contains

Protein	-	0.7 gm
Fat	-	0.1 gm
Carbohydrate	-	3.4 gm
Vitamin C	-	15 mg
Thanic	-	0.08 mg
Carolin	-	3.00 mg etc.

Besides these, mineral salts like calcium, phosphorus, iron, vitamin A and B are also richly available in Radish.

4. Curative Properties of Radish : —

Indigestion and Stomach problems : —

(i) Taking fresh radish with or without carrots and tomatoes eliminates acidity.

(ii) Taking radish with Sendha namak and black pepper sprinkled on it at meal time improves digestion and eliminates wind and acidity.

(iii) Taking juice of fresh radish, cabbage and tomato-cures flatulence.

(iv) Taking juice of fresh radish with little sendha namak twice a day cures stomach-ache and other problems of digestion.

(v) Taking the raw roots of Radish helps in digestion and increases appetite.

(vi) Taking Radish pieces (soaked for two days in mustard seeds powder) brings back appetite.

Constipation : —

Taking fresh leaves of Radish with Kala namak cures constipation.

Urinary problems : —

(i) Taking 30-40 gms of fresh Radish juice eliminates irritation and pain while urinating and also cures stranguary.

(ii) Taking fresh leaves juice twice or thrice a day or juice of root of fresh radish is also useful.

Stones : —

(i) Taking 1 cup juice of radish 3 or 4 times a day and chewing its fresh leaves or taking Radish seeds water (35 gms seeds, which are inside the covering of the beans of radish, boiled in half litre water till it is reduced to half) for few days-helps in breaking stones and throwing them out.

(ii) Taking juice of fresh Radish helps in stopping the formation of Gall stones.

Hoarse Throat : −

(i) Taking about 4-5 gms of ground seeds of Radish with lukewarm water-clears the throat.

(ii) Gargling with lukewarm radish water also helps.

Mouth-blisters : −

Gargling with Radish juice mixed with water in the same proportion and little salt-cures it.

Foul Breath : −

Taking Radish juice with Mishri eliminates foul breath.

Lethargy : −

Taking pieces of white Radish and its soft leaves with lemon juice sprinkled on it eliminates lethargy.

Hiccough : −

Chewing soft leaves of 3-4 Radish cures hiccough.

Ringworm : −

Applying heated paste of seeds of Radish ground in lemon-juice on the affected part is useful in curing it.

Eczema, Itching and other skin problems : −

(i) Applying paste of freshly ground radish pulp for 1 hour before taking bath-is helpful in curing eczema.

(ii) Taking Radish with salad in meals with lemon juice sprinkled on it removes blood-impurities and cures itching.

(iii) Applying ground pulp of Radish on the face till it gets dried up before washing with cold water cures acnes on face.

(iv) Taking one Radish alongwith leaves or its juice regularly and applying the ground pulp on face-eliminates black spots and freckles.

(v) Massaging with Radish juice eliminates wrinkles.

Jaundice : −

Taking raw fresh Radish or Radish juice with sugar or Radish juice and sugarcane juice early in the morning-cures jaundice.

Worms : −

Taking Radish juice with little sendha namak and lemon juice after meals destroys worms and throws them out.

Arthritis : −

(i) Taking fomentation of steam of hot water of Radish soft leaves (boiled first in a closed utensil) eliminates swelling and pain.

(ii) Taking 1 tsp ground seeds of Radish with water is also useful.

(iii) Taking juice of Radish with sugar is useful.

Menstrual problems : —

(i) Taking 2-3 gms of ground seeds of Radish 3-times a day- regulates and relieves pain during menses.

(ii) Taking fresh leaves of Radish cures pimples due to lack of bleeding in menses.

Fire-burns : —

Applying paste of ground Radish pulp on the burnt portion helps in quick healing.

Eye-Care : —

Taking one Radish a day is very good for eye-sight.

Whooping Cough : —

Taking juice of Radish with sugar-cane juice in equal quantity and little ginger juice gives relief in this.

Insect-bite : —

(i) Applying juice of Radish or slice of Radish with salt (to be changed after 5 minutes) on the affected part eliminates poisonous effect of scorpion and

(ii) Taking radish juice after 3 or 4 hours relieves the affect of poison.

Piles : —

(i) Taking fresh Radish or 1 cup of juice with 1 tsp pure ghee twice a day helps in curing it.

(ii) Taking slices of Radish (kept in open with salt sprinkled on it overnight) empty stomach in the morning

or

(iii) Taking slices of Radish fried in ghee is also very useful.

Sexual weakness : —

(i) Taking Radish regularly helps in getting back lost sexual power.

(ii) Taking 2 gms of powder of seeds of Radish (Dry 50 gms seeds of Radish and powder them. Strain it) with butter or cream regularly for atleast 8-10 days eliminates sexual weakness.

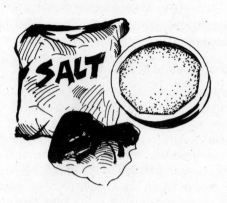

NAMAK (Salt)

1. Namak is known in different languages as :–

1.	Sanskrit	–	*Samudra, Vashira, Samudraja, Sagaraja.*
2.	Hindi	–	*Namak.*
3.	Latin	–	*Sodii Muras.*
4.	Bengali	–	*Karkacha Nun.*
5.	Marathi	–	*Meetha.*
6.	Telegu	–	*Upun.*
7.	Gujrati	–	*Dariyay Luna.*
8.	Sindhi	–	*Luna*
9.	English	–	*Salt.*

2. Description :–

Different varieties of salt are found. The most important available in natural form are five (i) sendha Namak (ii) Wid Namak (iii) Kaala Namak, (iv) Alkaline salt and (v) Sambhara Namak, **Sendha Namak**, the best of all types of salts is obtained from the mines underground. This is very tasty, digestive, light, appetiser, cooling, anti-phlegmatic, antibileous, anti-aciditic. This is easily absorbed in the body and in all the religious fasts this salt is used for preparing special food. **Vid Salt** is also obtained from the mines but artificial salt is also made. It is anti-phlegmatic, pain-reliever, anti-flatulent, digestive. **Kaala Namak** is tasty, carminative, digestive, releases wind and light.

Alkaline salt —procured from the salt of oceans, is sweet and bitter, digestive, appetiser, carminative, releases wind.

Sambhari salt—procured from Sambhar lake in Rajasthan, is light, anti-aciditic, very hot.

3. Chemical properties of Salt :—

Salt has combination of some natural elements : (i) Sodium (helps in curing aciditic gaseous effect and purifies blood) (ii) Chlorine (cleans the nerves, muscles and makes the body free from foreign elements) (iii) Calcium (helps in formation of bones and the body), (iv) Phosphorus-(helps in sharpening the mental faculties), (v) Iron — (helps in assimilating Oxygen and discharging Carbon-di-oxide in the body), (vi) Manganese — (helps in balancing salt proportion in the body), (vii) Potassium . (helps in giving strength to nerves, heart and liver), (viii) Copper- (adds to iron-contents in the body), (x) Sulphur-(clears blood and skin impurities), (x) Silicon— (strengthens eyes and ears), (xi) Magnesium — (provides general strength to the body), (xii) Fluorine— (strengthens the bones and controls gas and acidity). Apart from these salt is great tastemaker.

All these natural elements permeate not only in salts but all edible fruits and vegetable in different proportions.

Besides being an edible item-its uses are varied. Salt is used in making many detergents, chemicals and pesticides. It serves as means to solidify water in the ice-from. It is a disinfectant-its solution put in corners of wardrobes, boxes-clear off the moths. Salt is used as a stain remover-especially caused by ink.

4. Curative Properties of Namak :—

Indigestion stomach problems :—

(i) Taking 5 gm Black salt in hot water in the morning eliminates indigestion and improves appetite.

(ii) Taking Lavana Bhaskara Churna (made from the available 5 types of salt) with warm water after meals eliminates flatulence.

(iii) Taking the oozed water of onion pieces on which sendha Namak has been sprinkled after meals-is very useful in curing flatulence.

(iv) Taking ginger juice with little sendha Namak half an hour before meals improves appetite.

(v) Massaging the stomach with salt mixed in hot ghee-releases wind and cures stomach-ache.

(vi) Taking salt in hot water cures stomach-ache and also helps in easy movement of bowels.

Diarrhoea : —

Taking $\frac{1}{2}$ tsp. powder of sendha namak, Pipal and choti Harad (in equal proportion) with water after meals twice a day cures loose motions caused by indigestion.

Dysentry : —

Taking whey with little sendha namak with or after food-cures this.

Headache : —

(i) Keeping a pinch of salt on the tongue for 10 minutes and then drinking cold water-eliminates headache.

(ii) Rubbing little salt in pure ghee on the temples-gives relief in headache due to cold.

(iii) Putting one or two drops of salt water in the nostrils eliminates headache.

(iv) Smelling salt water (in 1 : 20 proportion) also is helpful in it.

Migraine : —

Licking $\frac{1}{2}$ tsp salt mixed with $\frac{1}{2}$ tsp honey brings relief in pain.

Baldness : —

Washing the head with salted water helps in hair-growth.

Dandruff : —

Washing the hair with salted water eliminates dandruff.

Eye-problems : —

(i) Washing the eyes with cold salted water (1 tsp salt in 1 kg. water) cures watery discharge, and eliminates swelling.

(ii) Washing the eyes with luke warm salted water-cures trachoma.

Dental problems : —

(i) Rinsing the mouth regularly with salted water-eliminates pain due to tooth-decay.

(ii) Applying strained salt mixed in mustard oil (kept in sun for one day) as toot-paste strengthens the gums and teeth and eliminates pyorrhoea.

(iii) Applying strained Kaala Namak mixed in Til oil as tooth paste-strengthens the loose teeth at their base.

(iv) Applying strained salt and peepal leaf powder with honey (in 1 : 3 proportion) as tooth paste for few minutes to let the saliva ooz out is also very useful in strengthening loose teeth.

(v) Applying finely powdered sendha Namak on the gums-relieves pain in gums and teeth.

Boils on tongue : —

Applying a paste made of white mustard seeds with sendha Namak and allow the saliva to ooz out eliminates boils on the tongue.

Hoarse Voice : —

Taking ground 10 gms. Ber (small red ones) with 2 gms sendha namak with honey 2-3 times a day cures hoarseness of voice.

Gargling with warm salted water also is useful.

Hiccoughs : —

(i) Drinking water with little sendha Namak gives instant relief.

(ii) Smelling a piece of jaggery with little sendha Namak sprinkled on it-or taking a piece of jaggery with water-stops hiccoughs caused by hot and spicy food.

(iii) Taking Kala and Sendha Namak with water and one lemon juice after meals is also useful.

Swelling and Pain : —

(i) Fomentation with potli of salt (on which little oil is applied)-heated on Tawa-gives relief in Bruise or sprain-pain and eliminates swelling.

(ii) Massaging the swollen part with pure ghee and salt mixture gives relief.

(iii) Rinsing mouth and gargling with salted lukewarm water eliminates swelling on neck and face.

(iv) Massaging around the joints with sendha salt roasted over fire in the til oil-eliminates swelling.

(v) Fomentatin with potli of salt-eliminates swelling due to Rheumatic fever.

Fatigue : —

Sitting in tub of lukewarm water with little salt-or putting feet in that water for few minutes eliminates fatigue and imparts freshness.

Cold and Cough : —

(i) Taking 1 glass boiled water with sendha namak, ground black pepper and turmeric-(Boil it till reduced to half) cures cold.

(ii) Dropping juice of Tulsi with little salt in the nostrils cures cold.

(iii) Massaging the chest with salted pure ghee gives relief in cold and helps in extracting the trapped phlegm.

(iv) Sucking a piece of salt gives relief in cough.

(v) Washing the nose or gargling or smelling the salted water- gives relief in cold and cough water-gives relief in cold and cough.

Asthma : —

Taking Sendha Namak and Desi Boora (1 : 4 proportion) with 100 gms warm water help in curing Asthma.

Bronchitis : —

Massaging salted lukewarm pure ghee on the affected portion eliminates the swelling in the bronchial chords.

Influenza : —

Taking paste of 5 garlic cloves and a little salt with hot Tulsi tea helps in eliminating the germs through sweat and urine.

Arthrites : —

(i) Fomentation with hot water and salt on the affected part gives relief.

(ii) Massaging the affected part with mustard oil and little salt (Kept in sun for 1 day) gives relief.

(iii) Taking bath with salted warm water is also useful.

Skin-problems : —

(i) Massaging the body with salted mustard oil removes dryness of skin.

(ii) Applying salted pure ghee in the navel cures dryness of lips and applying it on the feet and hands cures cracked feet and hands.

(iii) Applying ginger juice with sendha Namak on affected part eliminates acnes and pimples.

(iv) Taking juice or soup with sendha Namak, black pepper and lemon juice cures irruptions due to heat.

(v) Washing the affected part or taking bath with water in which husk of wheat and sendha Namak (in 10 : 1 proportion) has been boiled and then cooled regularly eliminates skin eruptions, cures itching and eczema.

(vi) Applying paste of salt and water on the affected part also help in curing eczema and other skin problems.

Vomiting : —

(i) Taking ginger and lemon juice with sendha Namak controls vomiting.

(ii) Rubbing salted ghee on stomach in clockwise direction is also very useful.

Excessive Thirst : —

Taking salted Shikanjavi or salted lime water 2-3 times a day quenches excessive thirst.

Stones : —

Taking sendha Namak or Kala Namak mixed in lime juice and water 2-3 times a day helps in dissolving the stones, which then pass out through urine.

Worms : —

Taking banana sprinkled with sendha Namak and lemon juice on empty stomach for 2-3 days kills and throws out the worms.

Piles :–

Applying salt on the fistulas is very useful in curing piles.

Bleeding :–

Taking a little salt gives instant relief in bleeding.

Cramps :–

Fomentation with potli of common salt and ground turmeric dipped in warm mustard oil on the affected part gives relief.

Menstrual Problems :–

Taking 2 gm of salt in warm water 2-3 times a day help in natural flow of blood in menses.

Malaria :–

(i) Taking $\frac{1}{2}$ tsp (for children) and 1 tsp salt (fried on Pan (Tawa) till golden brown) with warm water given empty stomach helps in curing Malaria.

(ii) Taking sendha Namak and Desi Boora (1 : 4 proportion) with warm water is also very useful.

Mumps :–

Gargling with salted water and fomentation with salted warm water eliminate swelling.

Effect of Poison or hangover of liquor :–

Taking 60 gms of salt in water induces vomitting and helps in throwing out poisonous substance.

Insect Bite :–

Rubbing the affected portion with salt after pouring some water and also taking salted water eliminates irritation, pain and swelling caused by the bite of poisonous insect.

Scorpion-Bite :–

(i) Rubbing the affected part with half tsp garlic juice mix with $\frac{1}{4}$ th tsp salt melts away the sting.

(ii) Dropping four drops of saturated solution (by dissolving 3-4 gms of salt in 100 gms of water) in the eyes/ears opposite to the side on which the scorpion has bitten is very effective in nullyfying the toxic effect.

Dog-Bite :–

Rubbing the mixture of ground garlic and salt over the affected portion eliminates the effect of dog-bite.

Canadian Doctors have opined that ladies, wishing to have male progeny should have more saltish food as compared to milk, cheese, butter etc. They should start taking more saltish food not only during pregnancy but 6 weeks before conception. Salt produces potassium and sodium in the body and have great effect on chromosomes, which determine the sex of the baby.

Dr. Jacks Lorren, renowned Doctor of Montreal (Canada), said that out of 296 ladies, who adopted their dietary habits according to his instruction, 265 ladies could have the sex of the baby according to their choice.

(*Note* : Intake of salt should be stopped in patients suffering from Hysteria, Epilepsy, High Blood Pressure, Kidney problems, arthritis, eczema, itching etc.).

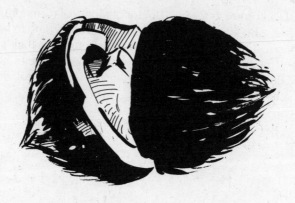

NARIYAL (Coconut-Palm)

1. Nariyal is know in different languages as : —

1.	Sanskrit	—	*Narikela, Langali, Skandha-phala, Sadaphala*
2.	Hindi	—	*Nariyal*
3.	Latin	—	*Cocosnusifera*
4.	Bengali	—	*Narikela, Narakola*
5.	Marathi	—	*Narali, Narala*
6.	Telegu	—	*Narikadama*
7.	Gujrati	—	*Naliyera*
8.	Tamil	—	*Tenna, Tenga*
9.	Sindhi	—	*Nariyal*
10.	English	—	*Coconut-palm*

2. Description : —

Coconut has enjoyed status of divine fruit. Hindus believed that Parashuram brought this fruit from Heaven. On Sharad Purnima Goddess of wealth Lakshmi is believed to come down on earth to see 'who on earth is awake after taking water of coconut'. Coconut tree is named as 'Jeevantaru' (life giving tree). It is really a great gift of nature to all beings. It is hard and tough outwardly but very soft and nice inwardly and symbolises a true Indian concept of ideal personality.

Coconut is a symbol of piety and prestige. The presentation of Coconut at auspicious occasions and religious and social functions. indicates advent of an event full of happiness, prosperity. It has become a part of Indian culture.

Even in temples coconut constitutes the most important part of the offering to Gods and Godesses & is a favourite 'prashad' to the devotees.

Coconut tree is grown all over India especially in Kerala, Karanataka, Bengal. It needs hot climate and damp soil with salt in it. So coastal regions and places near it are the most suitable places where coconut trees grow in abundance. It is 30-40 ft in height and it takes 8-10 years to yield its fruits.

Coconut fruit, though a bit heavy on the system, has cooling effect on the body. It is diuretic and gives instant vigour and vitality.

Its **raw fruit** has creamy delicious soft pulp and is carminative, digestive, antiflatulent, blood-purifier and a tonic. **Daab** (water of raw coconut) is cooling, quenches thirst, easily digestible, anti-billeous, antiphlegmatic, tonic for heart and recommended even for infants. **Ripe fruit** of coconut gives energy, removes aliments due to wind, bile and is a blood-purifier. The pieces of coconut are immune to any infection and so safe to consume.

Coconut oil is not only extensively used for black, soft and lustrous hair but also a cooking medium. Various tasty dishes, sweets, biscuits, etc. are prepared with coconut.

Besides the nutritive and therapeutical properties of Coconut fruit-its bark, shell, leaves, stem have different other uses. The **outer-covering** of Coconut is used in making many jute and other decorative items. Hard bristles on the shell are used for making brooms, brushes, door-mats, ropes, cushions of sofas, chairs. Dye is also made after burning the bristles. Its leaves are used for thatching the roofs of the huts. Its root is used as fuel to purify atmosphere.

3. Chemical properties of Coconut : —

The Kernel of Coconut contains

Protein	4.5%
Calcium	0.1%
Minerals	10.0%
Phosphoros	0.42%
Iron	1.7 mg per 100 gms.

It also has Vitamins A, B, C, D, and water.

4. Curative properties of Coconut : —

General Tonic : —

(i) Taking Daab (Coconut water) every day eliminates fatigue and gives vigour and strength to the body.

(ii) Taking dried coconut piece with milk is very good aphrodis for it helps in regaining lost energy.

(iii) Taking Coconut in raw form gives vigour and strength.

Insomnia : —

Taking Daab before going to bed induces sleep.

Worms : —

Taking Daab and pulp of green Coconut followed by 1 tsp olive oil for 2 or 3 days eliminates and destroys worms.

Stomach-ache : —

Taking Daab after food cures stomach-ache by eliminating acidity.

Piles : —

Taking 10 gms powder of burnt coconut shell bristles and jaggery with water-cures piles.

Headache : —

(i) Taking Coconut Kernel and Mishri before sunrise cures head- ache.

(ii) Massaging the head with the juice of coconut (dry coconut soaked in water and then juice extracted) cures headache.

Liver : —

Taking Daab water regularly-cures problems connected with liver.

Migraine : —

Dropping few drops of Daab in the nostrils eliminates pain.

Urinary Problems : —

Taking Daab water regularly cures stranguary, polyuria and other urinary problems.

Vomiting : —

(i) Taking 2 gms of burnt ashes of Coconut shell bristles with water stops nausea and vomiting.

(ii) Taking Daab water 3 or 4 times a day controls vomiting.

Nose-bleeding : —

Taking Coconut kernel empty stomach in the morning cures bleeding from nose.

Liquor hangover : —

Taking Daab water eliminates hangover due to liquor.

Itching and Abrasions of Skin : —

(i) Massaging with Coconut oil mixed with lemon eliminates itching.

(ii) Applying Coconut oil with little Camphor on the affected part-gives quick relief.

(iii) Applying Coconut oil with tomato juice is also useful.

(iv) Rubbing Coconut oil on the hands, feet, face makes the skin soft and eliminates abrasions caused by cold weather.

Stones : –

Taking Daab water is useful in breaking the stones and pushing them out.

Leucoderma : –

Applying Coconut oil with Camphor (in proportion of 5 : 1) on the affected part twice a day regularly is helpful.

Eye Problem : –

Taking Coconut kernel with jaggery daily for 7-8 days eliminates common eye-problems.

Pregnancy and post natal care : –

(i) Taking Coconut kernel with mishri during pregnancy helps in child's growth and easy delivery.

(ii) Taking Coconut oil with jaggery after delivery for 2-3 days gives quick relief in pain.

Poison of Rodent : –

Applying oil of an old Coconut piece with little radish juice on the affected part eliminates poison.

Fire-burns : –

Applying Coconut oil with juice of Tulsi leaves on the burnt part of the body gives relief.

Dandruff and Hair problem : –

(i) Massaging the scalp regularly with Coconut oil with camphor added to it eliminates dandruff.

(ii) Applying Coconut oil on hair-helps in checking greying and falling of hair and imparts lustre to hair.

Typhoid : –

Taking Daab water is very soothing in Typhoid.

Precaution : –

(i) Coconut should not be taken by persons suffering from cough or Asthma.

(ii) Excessive intake of dried Coconut-fruit causes constipation and flatulence.

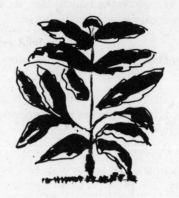

NEEM (Margosa Tree)

1. Neem is known in different languages as under : —

1.	Sanskrit	—	*Nimba, Arishta, Sarvatobhadrak, Ravi-priya, Shukrapriya Pitasar, Niyaman,*
2.	Hindi	—	*Neem,*
3.	Latin	—	*Azadirachta Indica,*
4.	Bengali	—	*Neemgachha*
5.	Marathi	—	*Kadunimba,*
6.	Telegu	—	*Veya*
7.	Gujrati	—	*Leemado,*
8.	Sindhi	—	*Nim*
9.	English	—	*Indian Lilac, Niba tree, Margosa tree.*

2. Description : —

Neem, the most favourite tree, is grown & found all over India. It has got 3 varieties (i) Ordinary Neem (ii) The sweet Neem and the (iii) Vilayati neem-known as Bakayan or Mahanimb; which have different inherent qualities. The ordinary Neem tree is 30-36 ft. high & provides a lot of shade to travellers. At the advent of spring the tree is full of fresh leaves and fruits (Nimboli). Its leaves are bitter but ripe Nimbolis are sweet in taste. The small lines on Neem leaves imparts to the tree a unique beauty.

Neem is cool and has soothing effect. It is antiseptic in nature. It is a blood and air purifier. It helps in eliminating digestive problems, cough, cold, fever and other physical ailments.

Every part of the tree-its rind, leaves, wood, flowers, fruits have great medicinal and therapeutic properties. Neem has contributed in manufacture of various Ayurvedic, Unani and Allopathic Drugs. The use of bark of neem purifies the blood. It is digestive, suppresses ill effects due to wind, bile and phlegm. The oil extracted from Neem is very useful for imparting energy and is a great antiseptic. The oil extracted from its ripe, yellow flowers-known as 'Margosa oil' is very beneficial for curing Arthritis, Leprosy, Leucoderma and other skin diseases. Neem soap is a great antiseptic, which cleans the body of all external impurities. Neem is an insecticide, which destroys and kills germs, insects. Dry Neem leaves kept in the cupboard or boxes protects the clothes, books etc. from worms and other insects. Neem's tender twigs used as tooth brush are very beneficial to keep gums and teeth strong and shining free from bad odour & pyorrhoea. Its wood is used for making furniture. Neem tree is a natural air-purifier, which wards off foul gases and gives oxygen.

3. Chemical Analysis : –

The Neem leaves are rich in (i) Protein (ii) Calcium (iii) Vitamin A.

Neem seeds contain oily sustance-known as Margosa or Neem oil-which is rich in sulphur.

Neem bark contains Iron, Phosphorus, Sugar, Sulphur in large quantity.

4. Curative Properties of Neem : –

Headache : –

Dropping one or two drops of juice of fresh Neem leaves in the nostrils cures headache.

Baldness : –

Applying Neem oil on the bald position preferably at night and washing the head in the morning stops the falling of other hair and helps in their growth.

Falling of Hair & Greying Hair : –

(i) Washing the hair with water (in which Neem and Beri or simple Neem leaves are boiled) stops falling of hair & helps the hair to grow & be black & lustrous.

This is also useful to kill lices in the hair (Precaution this water should not entire the eyes).

(ii) Applying paste of leaves of Beri & Neem in proportion of 2 : 1-on the head & washing after 6-8 hrs. stops hair falling and makes them soft and shining.

(iii) Applying Neem Tel-helps in stopping fall & greying of hair and makes them black and soft. (Grind Neem leaves with water and strain it. Mix Sarson Ka Tel & extracted juice of Neem in equal quantity and boil it on slow fire till all the water evaporates. After cooling store in a bottle for use).

(iv) Applying paste of Nimbolis of Neem & washing the head after 3-4 hours-helps in eliminating lices and improves growth of hair.

Ear-trouble : –

Taking the steam of boiled water having Neem leaves in it by the ear gives relief in ear-ache.

Dental troubles : –

(i) Using fresh Neem twig piece as brush for cleaning the teeth makes the gums strong, eliminates foul smell & cures pyorrhoea.

(ii) Use of Neem tooth powder (Dry the branch of Neem tree with leaves in shade-burn it. Grind it with little Pepperment, salt and cloves and then strain it through a cloth) strengthens the gums and teeth and checks foul smell.

(iii) Drinking and gargling with Neem water (in which fresh new leaves are boiled) stops dental decay and pain in the teeth.

(iv) Gargling with neem decoction (made with boiling of neem leaves, flower, nimboli, root and branchs in equal proportion) gives relief to tooth-ache by eliminating infection in gums.

Cough : –

Gargles with Neem juice mixed with lukewarm few drops of honey cures cough trouble.

Constipation : –

Rinsing the mouth with hot water in which 10 gms neem leaves have been dissolved early in the morning cures constipation.

Vomiting : –

(i) Taking Neem water (Grind 25 gms Neem Leaves mix it in 125 gm water and strain it) cures nausea and vomiting.

(ii) Applying paste of Neem flower ground with water on the navel portion-stops vomiting.

Digestive Problems : –

Eating 10 fully ripe Nimbolis daily with or after meals helps in curing indigestion.

Diarrhoea : –

(i) Heat inner bark of Neem tree on Iron Tava. Grind it nicely when burnt. Taking a pinch of this powder with curd helps in curing loose motions.

(ii) Swallowing powdered Neem seed and sugar with water controls loose motions.

(iii) Taking ground 10 leaves of Neem and Mishri with water checks diarrhoea especially in summers.

Dysentery :—

(i) Taking Neem decoction (prepared by boiling neem rind in double quantity of water) or 2 gm ground rind powder with water or honey juice in a day activates the system and controls dysentery.

(ii) Taking 10 gms. neem juice of leaves in the morning also helps in curing it.

(iii) Taking decoction of Neem leaves (Heat the juice of Neem leaves on fire Cool & strain it) cures dysentery.

Fatigue :—

(i) Chewing a few neem leaves helps in eliminating fatigue.

(ii) Eating Chutney of Neem leaves with little honey in it imparts energy and removes fatigue.

(iii) Chewing 5 leaves of Basil and 5 leaves of Neem with honey gives instant relief and energy.

Itching & other skin ailments :—

(i) Applying paste of Nimbolis ground with water or Neem oil on affected part cures itching.

(ii) Taking 20 gms of juice of soft fresh Neem leaves 2 or 3 times a day cures itching caused by impurity of blood.

(iii) Taking 30 gm of Neem juice (Soak ground Neem leaves and flower if available in water overnight and strain it) with honey cures all impurities of blood.

(iv) Applying paste of Neem leaves mixed with curd on affected part cures ring worm.

(v) Applying the Neem ointment (put a branch with green leaves in boiling mustard oil in a iron utensil. Move it with Neem stick until it gets thickened into ointment) on the affected part is very beneficial for all types of bowls, pustules.

(vi) Taking 10 gms of Neem tody (a type of secretion from certain Neem trees) cures all types of blood-impurities and checks skin diseases.

(vii) Taking this Neem tody regularly for 6 months to 1 year is very helpful in chronic cases of leprosy and other skin diseases.

(viii) Taking 5 gm juice of fresh Neem leaves and bathing with Neem water (water with Neem leaves boiled in it) helps in curing various skin diseases.

(ix) Swallowing 1 tsp powder of dried Neem leaves, Neem flower and Nimboli in equal quantity once in a day cures leucoderma.

(x) Taking fresh juice of Neem leaves regularly stops the pimples and acnes. Applying paste of Neem rind or Neem oil also cures pimples and acnes.

Digestive and stomach ailments : —

(i) Taking 10 gms of powder (made by grinding rind of Neem, dry ginger and black pepper-straining it through a fine cloth) with water in morning for 3 days cures acidity problem.

(ii) Taking ground 20 Neem leaves, 2 cloves, 3 seeds of Black pepper with little sugar-and water-twice a day for 2 to 3 days cures indigestion.

(iii) Eating 10-12 ripe Nimbolis daily with or after food activates digestive system and normal appetite is resumed. This cures flatulence.

(iv) Taking 3 gms of neem juice in ginger and mint juice 1 gm each, little Ajwain and kaala Namak and Sendha Namak after food cures digestive problems.

(v) Drinking Neem water (boil 100 gms of Neem leaves in 250 gms water and strain it) 2 or 3 times a day helps in regaining normal appetite.

(vi) Taking 4 gms of Churna (by grinding green but dry leaves) with water 3 or 4 times a day activates appetite and cures dyspesia.

Stones in Urinary Bladder : —

Taking 2 gm burnt ashes of Neem Leaves with water breaks the stones,which come out with urine. (Burn the leaves in a utensil after drying them in shade. Cover the utensil, After 4 hrs. grind the leaves).

Piles : —

(i) Taking 3-4 Nimbolis regularly helps in stopping excessive bleeding in piles.

(ii) Taking powder made of 3 gm inside part of the rind of neem with 5 gm of jaggery regularly cures piles.

(iii) Applying and rubbing about 5 drops of Neem oil on the haemorrhoids for 7-8 days helps in curing piles.

(iv) Taking powder of 10 Nimboli seeds, little Sendha Namak, Gur jaggery or Mishri with fresh water two times a day helps in curing piles.

Leucorrhoea : —

(i) Taking the juice of the rind of Neem with white cuminseeds checks leucorrhoea.

(ii) Drinking cow's milk with little Neem oil in it at night regularly cures this.

Menstrual Disorders : —

(i) Taking juice of 10 fresh Neem leaves and ginger juice in the same proportion with 10 gms water-eliminates and cures excessive pain during menses.

(ii) Taking paste of Neem leaves (Neem leaves to be boiled and ground) below the navel will check pain during menses.

Labour pains and delivery :—

(i) Tying Neem root in the waist of pregnant woman helps in early child birth. (caution-this neem root should be thrown away soon after child is born).

(ii) Taking Neem water (in which Neem leaves have been boiled for 15-20 minutes) will make the delivery less painful.

(iii) Taking juice of fresh Neem leaves on the 1st day of child-birth helps in contraction of uterus and works as an antiseptic.

(iv) Taking Neem water (water in which Neem bark is boiled) when thirsty for the 1st 6 days after child-birth is good for the mother's health.

Urinary Problems :—

(i) Taking 15 gm juice of tender branches of Neem with sharbat of unnab or sandalwood twice a day eliminates burning sensation or obstruction in the urinary passage.

(ii) Taking about 20-30 gms of juice of root of sweet Neem regularly cures urinary obstruction and burning.

Malaria :—

(i) Taking ground 2-3 leaves of Neem with black pepper on the day of the turn of Malaria helps in checking it.

(ii) Taking 1 gm powder of dried Neem leaves and Posat Doda with water, checks the inset of fever (on its turnday).

(iii) Taking 60 gms ground neem leaves, 4-5 black pepper seeds mixed with 120 gms of water-twice a day works as a preventive against Malaria.

(iv) Massaging the scalp and hair with Neem oil is also helpful.

Chronic Fever :—

Taking Neem water (boil 500 gm water with 21 Neem leaves and 21 black pepper seeds till the water is 125 gm) twice a day cures chronic fever.

Arthritis :—

(i) Massaging the swollen parts and other joints with Neem oil is very useful. (Boil 50 gm mustard oil and put fresh neem leaves in it till it become a bit black strain it and keep it in bottle).

Even cooking the food in this Neem oil is advisable for patients of Arthritis.

Paralysis :—

Massaging the affected protion with oil extraced from the seeds of Neem invigorates the dead muscles and tissues.

Diabetes :—

Taking decoction of rind of Neem (40 gms of the rind of neem to be boiled in 100 gm. water till 30 gm. is left Strain it) in the morning before breakfast eliminates sugar count in the urine.

Jaundice : —

(i) Taking 10 gms ground Neem leave, 4-5 Black pepper seeds & sugar with water in the morning regularly helps in eliminating the disease.

(ii) Taking ground Neem leaves and sugar mixed with water after heating it a little cures the disease.

Asthma : —

Taking 25-30 drops of oil extracted from seeds of Neem in bettle leaf gives great relief in Asthma.

Blister in the mouth : —

Applying Neem tel on the blisters with cotton cures them.

Sore throat : —

Gargling with lukewarm juice of Neem leaves and water cures soreness of the throat. 5 drops of honey and 2 drops of ginger juice may be added to extract the phlegm and eliminate the infection.

Heart-ailments : —

(i) Taking 10 gms juice of Neem leaves, ground cumin-seeds, mint and Kaala Namak-twice a day with lots of water intake during the day eliminates the burning sensation around the heart region.

(ii) Taking Neem Chutney with meals is very useful for controlling bile and stopping burning sensation.

(iii) Taking $\frac{1}{4}$ tsp. of ground seeds of Bakayan tree twice a day with water strengthens heart muscles and dissolves cholestrol.

Nose-Bleeding : —

(i) Applying paste of Neem leaves with little Ajwain on the temple stops bleeding.

(ii) Drinking juice of Neem leaves like Namkeen sharbat especially in summer is a preventive to those who suffer from nose-bleeding.

Poisonous Insect-bite : —

Chewing fresh Neem leaves with or without little salt and pepper helps in eliminating poison.

Worms : —

(i) Giving 3-4 drops of Neem tel to children and 5 to 6 drops to adults helps in killing the worms in intestines.

(ii) Taking 2 tsp fresh Neem leaves juice with 1 tsp honey kills the worms

(iii) Taking the paste of 1 tsp of juice of fresh Neem leaves with a little Heeng in it kills the worms.

Smallpox-Chicken pox etc. : –

(i) Munching boiled Neem leaves or 7 rednascent Neem leaves with 4-5 black pepper seeds works as a preventive against small pox, chicken pox.

(ii) On being afflicted-Neem twigs should be hanged on all room's entry and exit. (b) spread Neem leaves on the bed of the patient and change it twice in a day (c) give water with little juice of fresh leaves to the patient or water with Munakkas soaked in it (d) In case of burning sensation-the froth of juice of fresh leaves (which emits froth after whipping) may be applied on the boils.

(e) the patient may be fanned with Neem twig with leave.

(iii) After getting cured taking bath with Neem water and applying Neem. oil on the spots helps in quick healing of the spots.

Thus Neem tree, due to its innumerable uses and great therapeutic value in elimination of diseases is considered a treasure house of various medicines and can be used and enjoyed by one and all.

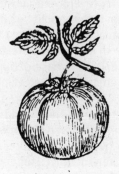

NEEMBU (Lemon)

1. Lemon is known in different languages as : –

1.	Sanskrit	–	*Nimbuka, Jambira*
2.	Hindi	–	*Kagazi Nimbu, Jambhiri Nimbu*
3.	Latin	–	*Lemonum Acidum*
4.	Bengali	–	*Kagaji Lebu, Pati Lebu, Jamira Lebu*
5.	Marathi	–	*Kagadi Limbu, Ida Limbu, Sakhar Limbu*
6.	Kannad	–	*Kachile Nimbu*
7.	Telegu	–	*Nimba-Pandu*
8.	Gujrati	–	*Kagadi Limbu, Khanta Gol Limbu*
9.	Tamil	–	*Elumichhai*
10.	Sindhi	–	*Leemu*
11.	English	–	*Lemon*
12.	Botanical Name	–	*Citrus Medica.*

2. Description of Lemon : –

The botanical name of Nimbu – 'Citrus Medica' clearly indicates its medicinal properties. Lemon tree is short in height & has oval leaves. There are different varieties of Lemon as Kagazi, Sharbati, Jambiri, Bijora etc. & is grown all over India.

Lemon is used with meals throughout the year in salads, drinks etc. but is particularly useful in rainy season as it supppresses bile.

Lemon Juice is sour in taste, quenches thirst, helps in digestion, increase perspiration, cleans Kindneys, acts as diuretic, cures diseases of elementary canals, purifies blood, imparts strength to the heart and controls bile, cough and wind.

3. Chemical Composition : −

1. Juice of Lemon is rich in Vitamin C
2. Citric-acid 7-10%
3. Phosphoric Acid
4. Folic Acid
5. Sugar
6. Calcium
7. Hesperedin type of Glucocide 5-8%
8. Vitamin B
9. Vitamin A
10. Potassium
11. Magnassium

4. Curative Properties of Lemon : −

Digestive Problems : −

Lemon juice taken early in morning with lukewarm water helps in comfortable cleansing of bowels & thereby increases the appetite.

Running Cold : −

Lemon juice taken in warm water with little salt helps in curing running nose.

Nausea : −

Lemon juice taken with little salt (black), powdered black pepper, Jeera and Ajwayan in glass of water relieves nausea.

Headache : −

Lemon juice taken in tea (without milk and sugar) relieves headache.

Obesity : −

Lemon-juice taken in lukewarm water early in the morning reduces obesity.

General Tonic : −

(i) Lemon-juice in fresh water with honey strengthens body and heart and tones up the muscles.

(ii) Taking pickle of lemon and unripe Black Pepper seeds helps in digestion & strengthens the body & muscles.

Urinary Problem : −

Fill the two pieces of lemon with little 'Kalami Shora' & heat it on slow fire. Take out its juice Rubbing it around the naval helps in passing out urine.

Diarrohea : −

(i) Lemon juice with tea (without milk & sugar) checks diarrohea.

(ii) Juice of one lemon in 300 gms water taken four or five times a day cures diarrohea.

Baldness :—

A paste of lemon seeds applied on the scalp cures baldness.

Small-pox :—

Taking lemon juice mixed with Gur (jaggery) helps in preventing small-pox.

Piles :—

Paste of lemon leaves with little sugar taken early in the morning checks piles.

Enlarged Liver :—

1 litre Nimbu juice, 100 gms Gingar juice, 10 gm salt, 20 gm Jeera, 5 gm Heeng.

Roast Jeera and Heeng. Powder them & mix with salt, juice of Lemon and ginger. Preserve in a bottle. Administration of this preparation 3 gm to 8 gm early in the morning helps in curing enlarged liver, increases appetite and cures all digestive problems.

Enlarged Spleen :—

(i) Taking Lemon juice (10 gm) mixed with onion juice (6 gms) morning and evening helps in curing enlarged spleen.

(ii) Taking lemom-pickle is also very good.

Blisters in mouth :—

Taking lemon juice either in soda, or juice of orange or pomegranate cures blisters in mouth.

Cholera :—

Taking lemon juice in glass of water mixed with Mishri in morning and afternoon prevents cholera.

Bleeding from Nose :—

(i) Putting fresh lemon juice with dropper in the nostrils helps in controlling the blood-flow.

(ii) Paste lemon juice mixed with Barley flour applied on the forehead once or twice helps in controlling blood-flow from nose.

Throat Problems :—

Taking hot lemon-juice with honey helps in curing throat problems.

Jaundice :—

Mix Nimbu juice (1 tola), Khanda (2 tola) Meetha Soda (4 Ratti), Nausadar (2 Ratti) with water (10 tolas) Taking it morning and evening helps in curing jaundice.

Dandruff, Hair Problems :—

Applying lemon juice mixed with Multani Mitti or Besan on the head & washing the hair 3 or 4 times checks dandruff, falling of hair and itching on the scalp.

Cosmetic Properties of Lemon :—

1. Cut a lemon in 2 pieces Rub soap on it early in morning. Apply & rub it on face and wash it with warm water. It helps in removing spots on face and imparts lustre.
2. Cut a lemon in 2 pieces & rub 10 gm Nausadar on these pieces with hand. When Nausadar gets absorbed then rub the pieces on tlhe face. It removes spots on face and gives a natural glow to the face.
3. Taking bath with hot water mixed with juice of 2 lemons softens and beautifies the skin.
4. Applying lemon juice mixed with Glycerin (equal quantity) and little Gulab-Water on face, hands and other parts of the body cleanses dirt, cures cracks and imparts natural glow and softness.
5. Brushing teeth with lemon-juice helps in eradicating foul smell and imparting sparkle to teeth.
6. Applying lemon-juice to hair before washing them makes hair soft and lustrous.
7. Applying on the head paste of one lemon juice mixed with 200 gm. Besan, 1 spoon mustard oil in 200 gm. water & then washing after some time imparts natural lustre and softness to hair.

The leaves of Lemon tree equally beneficial —

(i) Chewing 3-4 leaves 3 times a day helps in curing cough, bile & vomitting.
(ii) Taking paste of leaves mixed with sugar early in the morning cures diarrohea, dysentry & even piles.
(iii) Inhaling the smell of burnt dry leaves cures hiccough and headache.
(iv) Burning dried leaves in room helps in repelling mosquitoe and insects.

Lemon as stain-removes :—

Marble-slabs, Brass and Copperwares can be cleaned with lemon juice mixed with little salt.

Silver and gold ornaments can be cleaned with Lemon juice with Reetha solution.

Paleness of white clothes can be washed out by lemon juice mixed with little vinegar.

Old shoes can be cleaned & softened by rubbing them with peel of lemon.

Crockery and glass utensils, if washed with soap water with little lemon-juice, becomes sparking.

Applying Lemon-juice on hands eliminate foul smell due to garlic, onion, kerosene & also oil or grease on hands.

Murabba, Pickles and other tasty Preparation of Lemon : —

Murabba — Take large size Kagazi Nimbu Peel them slightly & prick them with a knitting needle. Boil them for a short time in lime water. After cooling them put them in thick sugar syrup.

Pickles — Take 1 kg lemon, 300 gm. salt, little Black Pepper, Jeera, Red Chillies; 10-15 Cloves, Soak lemon in water for a short time. Wipe them properly. Cut lemon it with partially into 4 segments & fill above mixture. Keep it in a jar covered with cloth in the sun for 5 – 6 days.

Note — Sugar or Jaggery can be added afterward according to taste.

Lemon-Chops — 500 gm, 300 gm potatoes, peas, Cauliflower, green chillies, garma masala, salt, pepper & Besan. Cut the lemon into pieces. Grate the Cauliflower mix it with boiled potatoes, & boiled peas, & other masalas. Wrap the lemon piece with this paste & dip it in Beasn. Then fry it. These lemon chops are very delicious and tasty & don't require any other Chatni with it.

Lemon is easily available at all times, at all places & is within reach of rich, poor alike. It is a gift of nature to mankind to keeping them healthy, smart & beauitful.

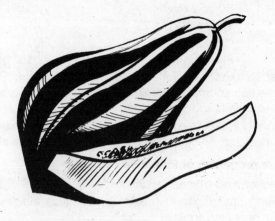

Papita (Papaya)

1. Papita is known in differentlanguages as : –

1.	Sanskrit	–	*Chirbhita, Nalikadala*
2.	Hindi	–	*Papita*
3.	Latin	–	*Carica Pappya*
4.	Tamil	–	*Pappali, Poppayi*
5.	Sindhi	–	*Papayo*
6.	English	–	*Papaya*

2. Description : –

Papita is grown all over India mostly in parts having hot climate with lots of rain. Papita of Hyderabad and Bihar is especially famous for its taste. The tree is of medium height. Its trunk is straight without any branches and it has an umbrella type of growth at the top, which bears fruits ranging from $\frac{1}{2}$ kg to 2 kg in weight. Every part of Papita has medicinal value.

Papita is an appetiser, digestive, antiphlegmatic, carrninative, diuretic, antiflatulent, vermifuge, pyreutic and a general tonic.

3. Chemical Properties of Papita : –

Papita contains :

Water	–	89.6%
Carbohydrates	–	9.5%

Proteins	–	0.5%
Ether extract	–	0.1%
Mineral Salts	–	0.4%
Calcium	–	0.01%
Phosphorus	–	0.01%

Its pulp also has Malic, Tartaric and Citric Acid, Resins, Pepen and sugar. The fruit is a rich source of vitamins, 100 gms of pulp has 3000 I.U. Vitamin A,130 mg-vitamin C and 56 calories.

The milk of Papita tree is very rich in 'Papain' - a digestive enzyme very useful as medicine. All other parts of Papita tree and fruit also have it.

4. Curative properties of Papita : –

Indigestion and stomach problems : –

(i) Taking ripe papita in breakfast eliminates indigestion, flatulence, acidity and increases appetite.

(ii) Taking water in which powdered dried leaves are soaked overnight is also useful.

Diarrhoea : –

Taking boiled raw Papita cures chronic diarrhoea.

Eczema, Ring worm, Itching : –

(i) Applying fresh juice of raw Papita on the affected part cures it.

(ii) Taking Papita regularly also is useful.

Freckles and other blemishes of skin : –

(i) Applying pulp of ripe Papita as ubtan on the affected part $\frac{1}{2}$ hour before bath eliminates freckles and other blemishes of skin and imparts natural glow and lustre.

(ii) Applying fresh juice of raw Papita is also useful especially for pimples.

(iii) Eating ripe Papita daily is also recommended.

Dandruff : Massaging pulp of Papita on the head 10 minutes before washing the hair eliminates dandruff.

Tonsilitis : –

Gargling with water in which little juice of Papita is mixed- cures tonsils.

Milk in breasts : –

(i) Taking ripe Papita daily helps in getting sufficient milk for the child.

(ii) Taking vegetable of raw Papita is also useful.

Menstrual problems : –

(i) Taking ripe Papita daily regulates menses.

(ii) Taking few seeds (powdered) with water is also useful.

High Blood-pressure : –

Taking ripe Papita half an hour before breakfast checks high blood-pressure.

Liver and Spleen : –

(i) Taking vegetable of raw Papita controls enlargement of liver and spleen of children.

(ii) Taking pickles of raw Papita or eating ripe Papita is also useful.

(iii) Swallowing $\frac{1}{2}$ tsp ground dried seeds of Papita with water and little salt two times a day also is useful.

Jaundice : –

(i) Taking 10-12 drops of raw Papita juice on 1 Batasha for 10-15 days helps in curing Jaundice.

(ii) Taking ripe Papita daily is also recommended.

Fever : –

Taking boiled water of Papita leaves eliminates fever.

Filaria : –

Tying poultice of Papita eliminates swelling.

Piles : –

(i) Taking ripe Papita in afternoon helps in curing piles.

(ii) Applying the juice of raw Papita on fistulas regularly also helps.

Worms : –

Taking $\frac{1}{2}$ tsp ground seeds of Papita with water for 3-4 days help in extraction of worms.

Stranguary : –

Taking ripe Papita regularly eliminates urinary problems.

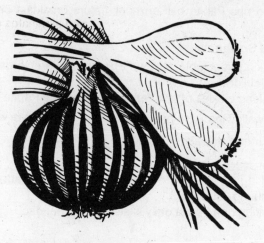

PYAJA (Onion)

1. Onion is Known in different languages as : —

1.	Sanskrit	—	*Palandu*
2.	Hindi	—	*Pyaja*
3.	Latin	—	*Allium cepa*
4.	Bengali	—	*Peyaja*
5.	Marathi	—	*Kanda*
6.	Kannada	—	*Irulli*
7.	Telegu	—	*Yarrulli*
8.	Gujrati	—	*Dungri*
9.	Tamil	—	*Vangain*
10.	Sindhi	—	*Basar*
11.	English	—	*Onion*

2. Description : —

Onion Plant is grown all over India. The edible part is the bulb which remains underground and fibrous roots come out of it. The plant is 3-4 ft high with cylindrical, conical & succulent leaves which are also edible. The bulb (onion) is of different colours white, red & pale. White onion is the most useful medicinally but the commonly used is the red variety. Its taste is sweet and pungent. It is an appetiser and helps in digestion of food.

3. Its Chemical Composition is :—

(i)	Protein	—	1.2 to 1.4 gm	per cent
(ii)	Fat	—	0.1	,,
(iii)	Mineral salt	—	0.4– 0.7	,,
(iv)	Carbohydrates	—	11.6–13.2	,,
(v)	Calcium	—	0.04–0.18	,,
(vi)	Phosphorous	—	0.05–0.06	,,
(vii)	Iron	—	0.8–1.2 mgm	,,
(viii)	Vitamin B	—	40 lu	,,
(ix)	Vitamen C	—	11.00 mgm	,,
(x)	Sugar	—	12.00	,,
(xi)	Crotene	—	55 lu	,,
(xii)	Thymin	—	120 mcgm	,,
(xiii)	Niacin	—	5 mcgm	,,
(xiv)	Water	—	87 mg	,,
(xv)	Also Evaporative oil of onion contains traces of sulphur.			

4. Curative Properties of Onion :—

Onion is a source of energy & acts as a stimulant, increases vigour & vitality, acts as an expectorant and diuretic, slows the heart beat, prevents flatulence and dyspepsia. It is useful in various diseases.

Insomnia :—

One teaspoon of onion juice mixed with milk or honey taken at bed-time induces sleep.

Cough :—

Onion juice mixed with ginger juice & honey act as an expectorant.

Cold :—

Eating raw onion or applying onion juice on the forehead helps in controlling cold.

Asthma :—

Onion juice mixed with ginger juice black pepper & salt or ground onion with honey helps in controlling Asthma and problems of throat, tonsils and lungs.

Tuberclosis :—

Intake of raw onion prevents and guards the attack of T.B. germs & also helps in eradicating T.B.

Pain in Ears :—

2 to 3 drops of lukewarm onion juice cures the pain in ears.

Eyes :—

One drop of onion diluted with rosewater helps in improving the eyesight and eliminates eye ailments.

Hysteria :—

Unconsciousness due to Hysteria is cured by making the patient smell onion or by rubbing his feet with crushed onion.

Cholera :—

(i) One cup of onion juice mixed with juice of one lemon, one teaspoon of ginger juice, pinch of Salt (table salt or Kaala Namak) given in four equal doses in a day prevents Cholera

(ii) One teaspoon of onion juice with little salt given two hourly or one spoon of onion juice mixed with juice of mint leaves given every hour helps in cholera.

Jaundice :—

Small onion cut into four pieces soaked in vinegar or lemon-juice taken with salt & black pepper twice a day helps in curing jaundice.

Urinary Problems :—

Onion juice taken in hot water acts as diuretic.

Stone (Pathari) :—

Onion juice mixed with sugar (sharbat) helps in braking the stone.

Diarrhoea :—

Applying paste of onion on navel region helps in curing diarrhoea.

Blood from the nose :—

Few drops of onion juice put in the nose helps in stopping bleeding from the nose.

Skin-diseases :—

(i) Onion mixed with turmeric powder and mustard oil, heated on fire into a paste and applied on bowl and abscess, helps in draining out pus.

(ii) One-fourth cup of onion-juice mixed with one cup of water used for washing the wounds & bowls etc. and applying a dressing of the same acts as a disinfectant and removes itching.

Heat-stroke :—

(i) In summers eating of raw-onion prevents heat stroke.

(ii) Applying the onion paste on the feet counteracts the effect of heatstroke.

Intoxication :—

Onion juice reduces the effect of over- intoxication.

Menstrual Disorders :—

Onion made into a curry with condiments or onion juice mixed with Gur taken regularly helps in curing menstural disorders.

Acne :—

(i) Applying onion-juice on acnes cures the overgrowth (Massa).

(ii) Seeds of onion ground and mixed with milk beautifies the skin by cleansing the spots etc.

(iii) Rubbing paste of onion with lime helps in removing the small overgrowth of skin.

Insect-bite :—

Applying paste of onion helps in curing the poisonous effect of bite of insects like honey-bee, yellow jacket, scorpion etc.

Baldness :—

Rubbing onion juice on the bald area of the head helps in new growth.

Dental Problems :—

Eating raw-onion prevents bacterial growth in the mouth, stops dental decay, helps in curing dental problems.

Arthritis :—

Rubbing of onion juice with oil of sesamum cures arthritis. Besides curative properties onion has other uses also.

Keeping of onion piece in the room is helpful to remove the smell of fresh paint in the room.

Keeping one onion in pocket is advised as preventing heat-stroke.

Tying of a piece of onion near the light dispels mosquitos, insects etc. coming in the room.

Keeping white onion prevents snakes from entering the house.

Onion is a boon and is like an 'Amrit-phala' for the labourers and poor class. They often eat chapatis with onion and salt only & are found healthy & free from various ailments from which rich people generally suffer.

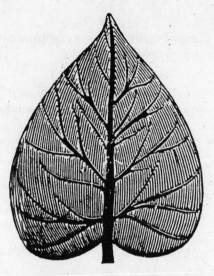

PAAN (Betel-leaf)

1. Pan is known in different languages as : −

1.	Sanskrit	−	*Jambuli, Jambulavalli, Nagavela*
2.	Hindi	−	*Pan*
3.	Latin	−	*Piper-betel*
4.	Bengali	−	*Pan*
5.	Marathi	−	*Nagavela, Pan*
6.	Kannada	−	*Nagara-valli*
7.	Telegu	−	*Tamalpaku*
8.	Gujrati	−	*Nagarbelana, Pan*
9.	Tamil	−	*Bettili*
10.	Sindhi	−	*Pan*
11.	English	−	*Betel-leaf*

2. Description : −

Pan is grown all over India and its Creeper is very attractive to look at. Its Pipal shaped leaves are whitish green or dark-green in colour. Many varieties of Pan are available depending upon different climatic conditions. Most popular among them are (i) Bengala (ii) Mahoba (iii) Maghahi (iv) Kapoori (v) Meetha (vi) Desi. Pan is extensively taken by Indians. It is a bit sour in taste but is a popular mouth freshner.

Pan is usually used as masticatory. It is stimulant, digestive, carminative, antiflatulant, anti-inflammatory, invigurating, antiphlegmatic, pain-reliever. It eliminates foul smell and is an antiseptic.

3. Chemical properties of Paan : –

(i) The leaves of Pan yield betel oil, which is light, aromatic and volatile. This betel oil contains terpene, betel-phenol and sesquiterpene.

(ii) It also yields a very volatile essential oil known as 'Chavicol'

4. Curative properties of Paan : –

Indigestion and stomach problems : –

(i) Taking Pan (prepared with Catechu, lime, betel-nuts, Ilayachi) after meals cures digestive problems and eliminates flatulence.

(ii) Fomenting the stomach (especially in case of Children) with heated leaf of Pan cures stomach-trouble.

(iii) Taking 2 tsp decoction of Paan (Boil 3 Paan with little blackpepper in 250 gm water and strain it) twice a day cures indigestion (especially good for children).

(iv) Putting the stalk of leaf smeared with oil in rectum (in case of constipation) helps in easy movement of bowels.

Headache :: –

(i) Applying ground paste of Pan on temples relieves headache.

(ii) Putting 1-2 drops of Pan juice in nostrils also eliminates headache.

Cold, Cough : –

(i) Taking clove in Pan relieves cold and cough.

(ii) Taking roasted Haldi piece in Pan or little Ajwain in Pan eliminates frequent coughing.

(iii) Keeping heated Pan (with Til or Arandi oil rubbed after heating Pan) in layers on the chest gives instant relief in coughing.

(iv) Taking 1 tsp Pan juice with little Golochana twice a day eliminates trapped phlegm in the throat.

(v) Taking Bengala Pan with a clove in it after meals expectorates the trapped phlegm inside.

Bronchitis : –

Applying heated Pan oil on the chest and covering it with cloth relieves bronochial congestion.

Inflammation of throat : –

(i) Taking Pan juice is helpful in eliminating inflammation of throat, layrnx and bronchi.

(ii) Gargling with 1-2 drops of Pan juice in 1 cup warm water relieves pain and inflammation.

Swelling :—

Keeping Pan leaf over the swollen part after heating it a little and tied with cloth subsides the swelling.

Diptheria :—

Inhaling the steam of 100 gm hot water with 3-4 Pan juice or gargling with it works as an antispetic.

Ulcers :—

Covering the affected part with Pan leaf is a ready dressing and cures foul ulcers.

Blisters in mouth :—

Chewing Pan with little camphor in it and spitting out frequently gives relief in blisters and also checks pyorrhoea.

Note : This Pan juice should not go in stomach.

Fire-burns :—

Tying Pan leaf on the burnt portion eliminates burning sensation and gives quick relief.

Gout :—

Keeping heated pan leaves on the affected joints and then tying with a cloth eliminates swelling in joints and cures pain.

Hoarse Throat :—

(i) Chewing the root of Pan creeper is very good for curing hoarseness of throat.

(ii) Taking Pan specially with Mullathi is very soothing to the throat.

Lungs Problems :—

Taking $\frac{1}{2}$ tsp Pan juice and $\frac{1}{2}$ tsp ginger juice with 1 tsp honey twice a day eliminates lung problems and strengthens them.

Preservative :—

Keeping Pan with green vegetables like mints, coriander leaves etc. makes them fresh for a longer time.

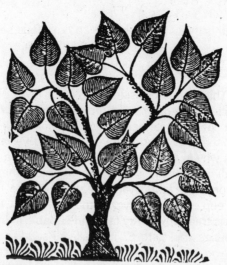

PIPAL(Popular leaved fig tree)

1. Pipal is known in different languages as : —

1.	Sanskrit	—	*Bodhidru, Pippala, Asvattha, Chala-patra, Gajasana*
2.	Hindi	—	*Pipal*
3.	Latin	—	*Ficus Religiosa*
4.	Bengali	—	*Ashvatha, Ashotha Gancha*
5.	Marathi	—	*Pimpala*
6.	Kannada	—	*Arali*
7.	Telegu	—	*Raichettu, Kulujubuichetta*
8.	Gujrati	—	*Pipalo*
9.	Sindhi	—	*Pipal*
10.	English	—	*Poupular Leaved Fig Tree*

2. Description : —

Pipal is one of the sacred trees of the world. Its Latin name Ficus Religiosa and English name 'Sacred Fig' — also bespeak its religious sanctity. In India especially it is considered to be a very sacred and respected tree. In Shrimad-Bhagwat Lord Krishna established the uniqueness (worthiness) of Pipal tree, where he says that "Among trees I am Ashwatha i.e. Pipal'. The world is called 'Urdhvamulo Ashvatha' i.e. Pipal tree having its roots in the sky according to Upnishads. Other Hindu sacred literature emphasize on its sanctity when they write that "Gods dwell on each leaf of

Pipal tree "All this indicates the purity and religious sanctity attached with Pipal tree.

The Pipal tree has a very long durability. The Pipal Tree, under which Budha got full enlightenment, is said to be 2500 yrs. old and is named as 'Bodhidrum'. This tree is considered to be a giver of mental peace and harmony. This is very strong and sturdy with roots spreading very deep in the earth. So it has great capacity to hold the soil and keep it well bound. Its leaves, of the shape of heart, are very soft and velvety. It does not have flowers, that is why in Ayurveda it is known as 'Guhya Pushpaka' - (having hidden flowers). It has fruits in abundance, which when raw are green and when ripe become little reddish and are sweet in taste. Its branches are thin, long flat and keep on moving even in the absence of wind. This is the best shady tree. This tree grows very fast and capable to shoot itself out of the walls of the houses, rocks etc. So it is called 'Asuddha' but it is believed that the Peepal tree grows – whereever the birds, who have eaten fruits of Peepal excrete. Thus this does not require elaborate planting arrangements.

The Pipal tree has apart from its inherent purifying properties something special in them. This is the only tree, which gives out oxygen not only during day but 'night' also. That is why sleeping under Peepal tree is advisable. This tree, moreover, has the capacity to stand amid the severest storms and earthquakes. This tree is almost without decay. It is always green and verdant in different seasons and climates. Its wood is used in making packing boxes.

As such all its parts-roots, stalks, fruits, leaves, branches, bark are very useful for healthy long life. It is diuretic in nature, blood-purifier, wound healer, an antiseptic, controller of wind, bile and phlegm and good for skin.

3. Chemical Properties of Peepal :–

Its bark contains 4% Tannin Acid, which has the power to destroy different types of insects and germs.

4. Curative properties of Peepal :–

Indigestion and other stomach ailments :–

(i) Taking milk in which Pipal is boiled, relieves wind.

(ii) Taking ripe fruit of Pipal regularly cures stomach ache and eliminates constipation.

(iii) Taking paste of soft leaves of Pipal with jaggery cures stomach ache.

Cough :–

Taking decoction of Pipal's bark with honey 3 or 4 times a day cures coughing.

Asthma :–

Taking powder of the seeds of Pipal with honey is useful in asthma.

Mental Weakness : —

Take 12-15 soft leaves of Pipal and boil it in Cow's milk on slow fire till it is dry. Store it in a bottle.

Taking 2 gm. of this medicine with cow's milk twice a day energises the brain and sharpens the memory.

Malaria : —

Taking ground Pipal powder with honey cures malaria.

Leucorrhoea : —

Taking few drops of Pipal milk in a Batasha followed by cow's milk two times a day cures leucrrhoea.

Blisters in the mouth : —

Applying powder of Pipal's bark on the blisters in the mouth cures them.

Vomiting, Hiccoughs : —

(i) Drinking the water with powder of Pipal bark in it cures vomiting & stops hiccoughs.

(ii) Burn the bark of the Pipal. When it stops emitting smoke, mix it in a glass of water. Taking this water stops hiccoughs.

Gout : —

Taking decoction of bark of Pipal with honey regularly morning and evening cures gout.

Mumps : —

Gargling with decoction made of Pipal gives relief in mumps.

Enlarged Liver : —

Taking 1 tsp of Pipal powder with $\frac{1}{2}$ tsp. of honey regularly gives relief in enlarged liver.

Swelling and Pain : —

Applying paste from powdered bark on the swollen part eliminates swelling and cures pain.

Obesity : —

Taking 1-2 tsp of powder of Pipal with honey in the morning reduces fat.

Wounds : —

Applying paste of soft leaves of Pipal is useful in healing wounds.

Bleeding : —

(i) Applying milk of Pipal stops bleeding and checks inflammation.

(ii) Applying the powder (obtained by rubbing Pipal bark against stone) cures wounds.

Pimples, Skin Cares : —

Applying milk of Pipal on the pimples cures pimples and imparts a natural glow to the face and makes the skin soft.

Quick Conception : —

Taking powder of the fruits of Pipal is helpful in quicker conception.

Gums, Teeth-Trouble : —

Applying juice of bark of Pipal on the gums and teeth cures dental pain and makes them strong and shining.

Piles : —

Taking juice of 10-15 fresh leaves of Pipal and one Karela for 8 to 10 days cures piles (even when blood is coming)

Menstrual Disorders : —

Taking Pipal leaves juice controls menstrual disorders.

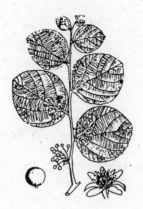

PHALSA (Asiatic Greevia)

1. Phalsa is known in different languages as : —

1.	Sanskrit	—	*Parusaka, Parusa, Alpasthi, Parapara.*
2.	Hindi	—	*Phalsa*
3.	Bengali	—	*Phalsa*
4.	Marathi	—	*Phalsa*
5.	Kannada	---	*Vattaha*
6.	Telegu	—	*Putiki*
7.	Gujrati	—	*Dharamanda*
8.	Sindhi	—	*Phalsa*
9.	English	--	*Asiatic Greevia.*

2. Description : —

Phalsa tree is found in all pars of India. This has medium height and has heart shaped thorny edged leaves growing on both the sides of the straight stem. Its fruits are small with a seed in side it. The fruits are attractive because of its mauve colour. These are available easily during summer.

Phalsa is sweet and little sour in taste. It is an energy giving tonic, destroyer of bile, heat and wind in the body, blood-purifier and antipyreutic. It keeps the body cool and purifies it of all the toxic elements.

3. Phalsa is rich in Vitamin 'C' and Iodine.

4. Curative Properties of Phalsa :—

Tonic :—

(i) Taking fresh juice of phalsa gives energy to the whole body.

(ii) Taking sharbat of phalsa in summers (Put 250 gms Phalsey in hot water, separate the seed-churn the pulp in sugar in mixie and sharbat with ice can be served) keeps away heat and makes the body healthy.

(iii) Taking Phalsey with sendha Namak daily in summer is refreshing and good for health.

Anaemia :—

Taking about 200-250 gms Phalsey with Sendha Namak eliminates Anaemia.

Its stones may also be crushed along Phalsey during summer for it eliminates the urinary problems and leucorrhoea in ladies.

Indigestion :—

Taking Phalsey with sendha Namak and black-pepper-increases appetite and cures indigestion.

Heart Problems :—

Taking juice of fresh and ripe phalsey with little sonth and jaggery strengthens the heart.

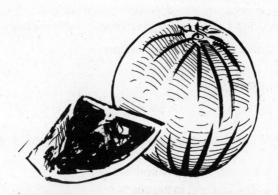

TARBUJA (Water-melon)

1. Water-melon is known in different languages as : —

1.	Sanskrit	–	*Kalinda*
2.	Hindi	–	*Tarbuja*
3.	Latin	–	*Citrulls Vulagris*
4.	Bengali	–	*Tarmuja*
5.	Marathi	–	*Kalingada*
6.	Kannada	–	*Kaude*
7.	Telegu	–	*Tarbujam Puccakaya*
8.	Gujrati	–	*Tarabuja*
9.	Tamil	–	*Tarbuja*
10.	Sindhi	–	*Chhahi*
11.	English	--	*Water-Melon*

2. Descripiton : —

The watermelon grows on a creeper in sandy soil near river or pond. The seed is sown 3" deep in the sand and at a distanee of 6" from each other during the month of February-March. The leaves are white & the flowers are of varied colours-white with black or green tinge. The fruit is green from outside. In unripe conditions it is white from inside and when ripe it becomes red or dark-red sometimes brownish or little dark. A Variety known as Matira is grown in Western Districts of Rajasthan as Jaisalmer, Jodhpur & Bikaner areas in the month of Oct-Nov. & becomes ripe by January or February. This variety is very sweet & tasty & can last for about one year, whereas the other variety can't last for more than 8-10 days. The weight of water-melon varies from $\frac{1}{2}$ kg to 10 kg.

Water-melon contains a high percentage of water & quenches thirst & is diureutic. Besides it gives energy, is digestive and very tasty.

3. Chemical Composition of water-melon : –

1. Water – 93%
2. Carbohydrates
3. Protein
4. Calcium
5. Phosphorous
6. Sugar
7. Iron – It is a rich source of iron
8. Cucurbocitrin is found in the seeds.

4. Curative Properties of water-melon : –

High-blood pressure : –

Juice extracted from the seeds, which contains cucurbocitrin, helps in dilating the blood-vessels, activates the Kidneys, brings down high blood-pressure and reduces oedema of the ankles. Juice is extracted by drying the seeds in shade & powdered. Two teaspoons of powder is put in 1 cup of boiling water for one hour. Strained & taken 4 times relieves high blood pressure.

Jaundice : –

Watermelon helps in curing enlarged liver and jaundice.

Heart Diseases : –

Thandai made with water-melon seeds mixed with rosepetal, melon seeds, blackpepper, poppy-seeds and almonds in water or milk is very nourishing and imparts strength to heart and brain.

Kidney Problems : –

One cup juice of water melon kept overnight in the open & taken with Mishri in the morning helps in cleansing the kidneys.

Heat-stroke : –

300 to 500 gms of watermelon taken with breakfast prevents & cures heat-stroke.

Stomach and digestive problems : –

Water-melon taken with little salt and pepper helps in removing constipation & other problems of indigestion.

Headache : –

One glass of juice mixed with Mishri taken before breakfast cures chronic headache.

Nausea : –

One cup of juice mixed with Mishri checks nausea and controls bile.

Mental disorders & Phobia : –

A syrup prepared in the following manner is to be taken regularly twice daily : – 2 kg watermelon crushed & boiled in $\frac{1}{2}$ kg water mixed with 4 kg. sugar, 25 gm. Cardamom (Illayachi powder); 20 gm. of Choti Pipal; 30 gm of Vamsalochan; 5 gm of Suhaga powder to be made into a thick syrup mixed with 100 ml. of Kewda.

Apart from the curative properties of the inner-pulp the outer shell with white portion of the pulp can be used far preparing vegetable, pickles, mixed with curd to form Raita & also sweet petha.

Precaution : Cut out open pieces sold in the market should never be consumed as they are most unhygenic & lot of dust & bacteria accumulate over them & its consumption may cause cholera and other diseases. Generally the best time to eat water-melon is one hour after lunch.

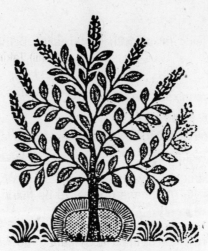

TULSI (Basil)

1. Tulsi is known in different languages as :—

1.	Sanskrit	—	*Tulsi*
2.	Hindi	—	*Tulsi*
3.	Latin	—	*Ocimum sanctum*
4.	Bengali	—	*Tulsi*
5.	Marathi	—	*Tulasa or Tulasi*
6.	Kannada	—	*Ereda-tulsi*
7.	Telegu	—	*Gappasa-chettu*
8.	Gujrati	—	*Tulsi*
9.	Tamil	—	*Tulsi*
10.	Sindhi	—	*Tulsi*
11.	English	—	*Basil*

2. Description of Tulsi :—

The botanical name 'Occimum Sanctum' (Latin) of Tulsi depicts that it is a sacred plant not only in India but throughout the world because of the outstanding medicinal and purifying qualities contained in essential volatile oils in the leaves, stem and the roots. It is grown and found almost all over the world. In India the plant of Tulsi is cultivated in almost every house & is also worshipped. Usually the plant is 1-2 ft high with fragrant small oval-shaped leaves, flat seeds red in colour, flowers blossoming on inflouroscence (manjari). White Tulsi & Black Tulsi are most commonly found although there are also Vana-tulsi, Rama-tulsi & Kappori Tulsi and Black Tulsi is the best as regards its properties.

Tulsi is mildly Pungent. It acts as an appetiser & helps digestion. It is beneficial to heart, suppresses excessive bile, cough and flatulence, removes blood impurities. All the parts of the plants i.e. seeds, leaves, shoots, flowers, stems and even the roots have medicinal value & are helpful in eradicating diseases.

3. Chemical Composition : –

Its leaves are particularly rich in fragrant volatile oil, from which Basil Camphor is made. It also contains very minute quantity of Mercury and has been reported to be useful in cancer patients in early stages.

4. Curative Properties of Tulsi : –

Malaria : –

Tulsi has been universally recognised as specific cure for Malaria and also acts as a preventive in checking Malaria

(i) Taking 1 tsp. Tulsi juice with little black pepper and honey taken 4 times a days cures Malaria

(ii) Decoction (Kaadha) made from roots of Tulsi mixed with sugar taken 3 to 4 times a day also cures Malaria.

(iii) Decoction made of 6-8 Tulsi leaves, one cardamom and little ginger taken regularly acts as a preventive against Malaria.

Cold & Cough : –

(i) Drinking Ten Tulsi leaves and 5 seeds of black-pepper to be boiled in one cup full of water till it is reduced to half cup & mixed with little Gur or Pure Ghee or Sendha Salt help in curing cold & cough.

(ii) 3 or 4 drops of Tulsi juice mixed with mother's milk helps in curing diarrhoea, cough, vomiting, indigestion of an infant.

(iii) Smelling of Powder of Tulsi leaves dried in shade helps in curing the running nose.

(iv) Heat 5 cloves and chew it with Tulsi leaves. It helps in relieving cough & cold;

(v) Taking 1 teaspoon of Tulsi juice mixed with little Pipal powder and double Mishri powder relieves Dry cough, fever & pain in chest

(vi) Taking 1 tsp of Tulsi juice mixed with little Powder of Saunf, Black pepper, Peepal and honey twice a day relieves cold & cough;

(vii) Taking juice of ginger and Tulsi in equal quantity mixed with honey cures cold & cough and acts as a general tonic.

Problems of Digestion : –

(i) Taking 1 tsp of Tulsi juice and ginger juice with water cures indigestion & relieves stomach- ache;

(ii) Eating Tulsi leaves with sugar or decoction of Tulsi leaves helps in curing diarrhoea;

(iii) Taking 1 teaspoon of juice of Tulsi leaves or Tulsi Juice mixed with powdered cardamom and honey relieves nausea & vomiting;

(iv) Taking juice of Tulsi, onion and ginger in equal proportion relieves biliary problems (excessive bile);

(v) Taking 1 teaspoon of Tulsi juice 3 times a day kills worms in the intestines;

(vi) Taking Tulsi juice with ginger, black pepper powder & Sendha Namak relieves flatulence and indigestion.

Headache : –

Applying Tulsi juice mixed with Camphor on forehead relieves headache.

Hysteria : –

Tulsi juice with little pepper kept in bottle and smelt everyday relieves attacks of hysteria and rejuvenates the brain.

Insomnia : –

Tulsi leaves and Ajwayan kept under the pillow induces sleep.

Unconsciousness : –

Drop of Tulsi juice mixed with a pinch of salt put in the nose helps regaining consciousness.

Ear Problems : –

(i) Drop of juice of Vana Tulsi put in ear helps in extracting of worms from the ear

(ii) In case of Pus and ache in the ear a drop of lukewarm Tulsi juice may be put.

Uterine Problems : –

(i) In case of excessive bleeding eat powder (Churna) made of Tulsi root with betel (Pan)

(ii) Tulsi seeds taken at the time of menopause relieves disturbances due to menopause,

(iii) For ensuring conception chew Tulsi seeds, or take powdered seeds with water or a decoction during periods

(iv) Tulsi-juice reduces labour pain.

Cholera : –

Taking tablets made of Tulsi juice with black pepper helps in Cholera.

Skin-diseases : –

Applying Tulsi juice mixed with lemon juice in equal proportion on the affected skin cures itching, pimples, blackspots, acnes and other skin diseases.

Asthma :—

Tulsi juice, ginger juice, and onion juice mixed with honey helps in taking out phlegm & relieves Asthma.

Leucoderma :—

Applying of Tulsi oil (Boil the ground Tulsi & its roots in $\frac{1}{2}$ kg water & $\frac{1}{2}$ kg oil on slow fire till whole of water evaporates. Mesh it thoroughly & filter it) thrice a days helps in curing boils, wounds & spots of leucoderma.

Rheumatic Pain :—

(i) Boil Tulsi leaves in water and pouring it on the affected part relieves rheumatic pain

(ii) Taking ground Tulsi leaves with black pepper and Pure ghee helps in curing the disease.

Hair-fall Grey Hair :—

Tulsi leaves and Amla Powder made into a paste with water applied on hair helps in strengthening the roots and darkening the hair.

Apart from its curative properties Tulsi is a highly beneficial & useful source of energy and general tonic for all.

(i) Swallowing five leaves with water early in the morning increases physical strength, mental faculties and imparts glow on the face.

(ii) 8 drops of Tulsi juice taken with water strengthens muscles and bones Tulsi seeds boiled in milk imparts vigour and vitality.

Tulsi leaves put in water purifies & makes it germ free.

Deep breathing (Pranayam) in the vicinity of Tulsi plants prevents many diseases.

Tulsi Plant purifies the polluted atmosphere. Followers of Vaisnava sect wear Tulsi rosary (mala) for physical and spiritual upliftment.

In short 'Tulsi' acts as a "Panacea and Preventive" in many diseases.

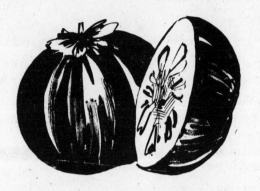

TAMATAR (Tomato)

1. Tomato is known in different languages as : —

1.	Hindi	—	Tamatar
2.	Latin	—	Lyso-perscion Esculentum.
3.	Gujrati	—	Tamatar
4.	Sindhi	—	Tamato
5.	English	—	Tomato

2. Description : —

Tomato is very popular vegetable in Europe and America and is nicknamed 'Love-Apple'. It is also grown in large quanties all over India. It has different varieties but most prevalent are 'Esculentum' (having fully grown big size) and Pimpinelipholium (having small size).

Tomato is a very tasty and nutrient vegetable. People relish it eating in raw as well as various cooked forms — Salads, Soups, Juice, Chutney, Raita and with different vegetables etc.

Tomato is digestive, carminative, diureutic, invigorating, germicidal, appetiser, stimulates blood-circulation and enriches red-corpuscles in the blood. It gives energy and strength to the muscles of heart and bones. It clears constipation, activates liver.

Tomato is a rich storehouse of Vitamins. The contents of Vit A,B, and C in Tomato are much more than in orange or grapes and is more useful than the latter. Eating 4 ripe tomatoes a day fulfils the entire requirement of vitamin

A in a human body. Vitamins in Tomatoes are not destroyed even when heated.

Tomato is rich in Iron, which is 2 times more than in eggs.

Thus tomato is a precious vegetable, which give a lot of energy and resistance to fight diseases. So eat Tomato and keep fit.

3. Chemical Properties in Tomato : —

100 gms Tomato contains

Water	—	93.1 gm
Protein	—	1.9 gm
Fat	—	0.1 gm
Mineral Salts	—	0.6 gm
Sodium	—	45.8 mg
Potassium	—	114.00 mg
Copper	—	0.19 gm
Sulphur	—	24.00 gm
Chlorine	—	38.00 gm
Thiamine	—	0.07 gm
Riboplaivin	—	0.01 gm
Nicotynic Acid	—	0.04 gm
Vitamin C	—	31.00 gm
Vitamin A	—	320.00 gm
Calories	—	23.00 gm
Calcium	—	20.00 gm
Oxalic Acid	—	2.00 gm
Magnasium	—	15.00 gm
Phosphorus	—	36.00 gm
Iron	—	1.08 gm

4. Curative Properties of Tomato : —

Tonic : —

(i) Taking one glass Tomato juice with little honey in breakfast- gives mental and physical strength and energy.

(ii) Taking Tomato soup before meals increases appetite, eliminates weakness and gives vigour and strength to the muscles.

(iii) Taking Tomatoes regularly strengthens the weak bones

(iv) Taking Tomatoes regularly with Sendha Namak or Jaggery sprinkled on it eliminates iron-deficiency during pregnancy.

Anaemia : —

Eating raw Tomatos and sucking its juice (after removing the seeds) helps in generation of blood and cures anaemia.

Indigestion and Stomach ailments : —

(i) Eating raw tomatoes with kaala namak and ground pepper sprinkled on it cures in-digestion and increases appetite.

(ii) Taking raw tomatoes or Tomato juice and lots of Spinach (Palak) eliminates Constipation and makes the bowels move easily.

Blisters in mouth : —

(i) Gargling with Tomato juice mixed with water cures blisters on lips, tongue and mouth.

(ii) Taking Tomato juice regularly is advisable for a person who suffers from this occasionally.

Nausea : —

(i) Sucking juice from a Tomato with Kaala Namak, Black Pepper and lime-juice sprinkled on it controls nauseating feeling.

(ii) Taking juice of Tomato and few Mint leaves with black-pepper Kaala namak and lime juice sprinkled in it relieves nausea.

Appendicites : —

Taking pieces of red ripe Tomtoes with finely chopped ginger and sendha namak before meals is good in appendicites

Eye troubles : —

(i) Taking raw ripe Tomatoes regularly improves eye-sight and eliminates eye troubles.

(ii) Taking tomatoes and curd combination as vegetable or syrup with meals is very helpful in improving eye-sight. (Tomato juice and curd in 2 :1 proportion mixed with either sendha namak, black pepper or jaggery).

Heart-Palpitation : —

Taking 1 cup juice of fresh Tomatoes mixed with little powder of the bark of Arjun tree for 15-20 days eliminates problem of palpitation of heart.

Skin-Ailments : —

Taking Tomato-juice regularly 2-3 times a day purifies the blood and cures skin-diseases.

(ii) Massaging the skin with Tomato juice mixed with the coconut oil is very effective in eliminating dryness of the skin and also cures itching.

Gum-bleeding : —

Taking 5 gms of Tomato juice regularly 3 times a day strengthens the gums and stops bleeding.

Black-spot, Freckles on Face : —

Applying the juice of Tomato by cottonwool (soaked in Juice) on the black spots or freckles on the face and washing after some time clears the spots and makes the skin glow.

Diabetes : —

Taking raw sliced Tomato with salt and pepper sprinkled on it reduces the sugar content in the blood.

(ii) Taking Tomato salad, Tomato vegetables and Tomato juice (like water) eliminates sugar content and cures diabetes.

Infantile Scurvy : —

Giving 20-25 gms juice of fresh ripe tomatoes thrice a day to children improves digestion and cures infantile scurvy.

Worms : —

Taking sliced fresh red tomatoes with sendha namak and black pepper sprinkled on it empty stomach destroys worms.

Piles : —

Taking fresh sliced tomatoes and raddish with Sonth, Kaala namak and roasted ground Jeera sprinkled on it with meals for 2-3 week cures piles.

Obesity : —

Taking fresh sliced tomatoes with onion, kaala namak, black pepper and lemon juice-sprinkled on it daily helps in eliminating fat from the body.

Fever and Thirst : —

Taking 50 gms juice of Tomatoes 2-3 times quenches the thirst caused by fever.

Tuberclosis : —

Taking 80-100 gms juice of Tomatoes with 1 tsp Cod-Liver Oil daily for 3 months gives strength and vigour and cures T.B.

Night Blindness : —

Eating Tomato by cutting it with teeth regularly eliminates night blindness (which is caused by lack of Vitamin A)

Gout : —

Taking Tomato and Bathua mixed juice 2 times a day eliminates and cures Gout.

Apart from these uses Tomatoes are useful as energy giving food item and can be eaten always with meals/breakfast etc.

Precaution : —

Tomatoes are harmful for patients suffering from

(i) Severe cough

(ii) Stone problems in sotmach, urinary bladder. Hence tomatoes should not be taken by them.

(iii) Too much intake of seeds in tomatoes may lead to stone- formation and so should be taken care of.

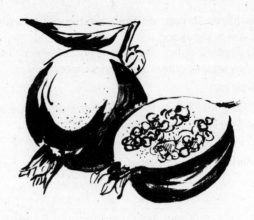

ANAR (Pomegranate)

1. Anar is known in different languages as :—

1.	Sanskrit	—	*Dadima, Dandabija, Lohita puspako, Karaka*
2.	Hindi	—	*Dadim, Anar*
3.	Latin	—	*Punica Granatum*
4.	Bengali	—	*Dadima*
5.	Marathi	—	*Daliva, Dalinva*
6.	Kannada	—	*Dadimba*
7.	Telegu	—	*Danimmchetta, Dalimkaya*
8.	Gujrati	—	*Dalima*
9.	Tamil	—	*Madai Chettaddi*
10.	Sindhi	—	*Anara*
11.	English	—	*Pomegranate*

2. Description :—

Anar tree is planted in almost all the parts of India but Anars of mountaneous regions of Northern India are especially very juicy and tasty. Anar grown in Kabul, Kandhara and Arabian countries is very popular.

The common adage "EK-Anar Sau Beemar" surely bespeak of its medicinal, therapeutic value and its nourishing and energy-giving contents. This fruit has lots of soft seeds of red or pinkish-white colour in it. The outer shell, however, is bit hard. Its roots, leaves, fruit, rind, seeds are all used for medicinal purposes.

Sweet Anar : –

Seeds are very soft, juice a bit pungent but very tasty and delicious. One of its famous variety 'Bedaana Anar' is very invigorating. Anar is digestive, carminative, enchances semen formation, activates memory, destroys disturbances caused by wind, bile, phlegm, improves formation of hemoglobin and is a blood purifier.

Sweet and Sour Anar is very tasty, usually used in preparing chaat of fruits but is acidic in nature **Sour Anar** is very effective in destroying wind and phlegm put creates acidity. So it should not be taken in large quantities.

3. Chemical Properties of Anar : –

Anar is rich in phosphorus, iron, calcium, and Vitamin C.

The rind and stem of this fruit have-Tannin (25-28%) mannite, pectin and an alkaline oily substance-Isopellectiercine.

4. Curative Properties of Anar : –

Tonic : – Taking juice of Anar regularly gives physical and mental energy and enchances blood-cells and improves blood circulation.

Indigestion and Stomach ailments : –

(i) Taking juice(15gm) or ripe sweet Anar with ground roasted cumin seeds (Jeera powder) and jaggery-twice a day-eliminates all stomach problems.

(ii) Taking seeds of Anar with powder of Kali Mirch and Sendha Namak sprinkled on it-relieves stomach-ache.

Cold and Cough : –

(i) Taking one tablet (Make the powder of rind of Anar tree with $\frac{1}{8}$ th Sendha Namak-mixed with little water to make tablets) 2-3 times a day relieves cough.

(ii) Taking tablet (Mix 20 gms rind of Anar tree-with 5 gm. Black pepper, 3 gms peepal, in syrup of 40 gms jaggery. Make small tablets about 2 gms each) 2 or 3 times with warm water dissolves trapped phlegm and is useful in cough and even Asthma.

Worms : –

(i) Taking decoction of rind of Anar destroys worms (Grind rind of Anar -25 gms-with 3 gms Palash seeds, 5 gms Vayavidang and heat it mixed with water on slow fire till the water is reduced to half, cool and strain it).

(ii) Taking 2 gm of dried ground rind of Anar and oranges-with Whey (Chacha) and little Kala Namak to taste-twice a day kills the worms.

Nose-Bleeding : —

(i) Pouring Anar juice in nostrils helps in checking bleeding.

(ii) Taking about 1 cup Anar juice with sugarcandy-2-3 times a day checks nose-bleeding.

Tooth-problems : —

Using the Anar flower powder (after drying the flower of Anar in shade-Grind them and strain) on teeth helps in curing bleeding gums.

Diarrhoea, Dysentery : —

(i) Taking powder of the rind of Anar stem (10 gm rind dried in shade and ground with 6 gm roasted Jeera and 10 gms jaggery) two times a day checks loose motions.

(ii) Taking $\frac{1}{2}$ cup juice (10gm rind of Anar dried and ground with 2 cloves and boiled in 1 glass water for 5 minutes) three times a day cures blood and mucus with motions.

Fever : —

Taking juice of Anar is very useful in fever.

Foul Smell in Mouth : —

Gargling with boiled water of rind of Anar helps in eliminating foul smell.

Heart Palpitation : —

(i) Taking 10-12 gms ground fresh leaves of Anar with 1 cup water 2 or 3 times gives relief.

(ii) Taking sharbat of Anar gives instant relief in palpitation of heart.

Intestine and Liver Problem : —

Taking Anar juice regularly cures all intestine and liver afflictions.

Piles : —

Taking about 6-8 gms of ground rind of Anar with water twice a day helps in curing piles.

Miscarriage : —

Applying paste of ground fresh leaves of Anar over the lower-abdomen-in case of feeling of pain-helps in controlling abortion or miscarriage.

Menstrual Problems : —

Taking 1 tsp ground dried rind of Anar with water twice a day stops excessive bleeding.

Leucorrhoea : —

Taking ground 20 gms fresh leaves of Anar with ground blackpepper in 1 cup of water-twice a day-controls leucorrhoea.

Night-discharge : −

Taking 3-4 gm ground dried rind of Anar with water twice a day regularly eliminates night discharge.

Polyuria : −

Taking 5 gm ground dried rind of Anar with fresh water morning and evening

or

Taking Anar flower (dried in shade) with honey twice a day cures too much urinating tendency.

Lices : −

Applying a paste of dried ground rind of Anar to the hair for half an hour before wash-clears off all the lices.

Beauty treatment : −

Applying the paste of dried ground rind of Anar mixed with Gulabjal and leaving it for sometime before wash eliminates spots, freckles on the face, improves the complexion, and makes the skin soft and lustrous.

Jaundice : −

Taking 10 gms of Anar juice (kept in a iron utensil overnight in open but covered with a thin cloth) with Mishri next morning regularly-helps in curing Jaundice.

HEALTH BOOKS

Yog Guru Sunil Singh
- Healing through Yoga — 75.00

Dr. Ashok Gupta
- Naturopathy for better health — 75.00
- Juice Theraphy for better health — 75.00

David Servan Schreiber (Guerir)
- The Instinct to Heal — 195.00
  (Curing stress, anxiety and depression without drugs and without talk therapy)

M. Subramaniam
- Unveiling the Secrets of Reiki — 195.00
- Brilliant Light — 195.00
  (Reiki Grand Master Manual)
- At the Feet of the Master (Manal Reiki) — 195.00

Sukhdeepak Malvai
- Natural Healing with Reiki — 100.00

Pt. Rajnikant Upadhayay
- Reiki (For Healthy. Happy & Comfortable Life) — 95.00
- Mudra Vigyan (For Health & Happiness) — 60.00

Sankalpo
- Neo Reiki — 150.00

Dr. Shiv Kumar
- Aroma Therapy — 95.00
- Causes, Cure & Prevention of Nervous Diseases — 75.00
- Diseases of Digestive System — 75.00
- Asthma-Allergies (Causes & Cure) — 75.00
- Eye-Care (Including Better Eye Sight) Without Glassess — 75.00
- Stress (How to Relieve from Stress A Psychlogical Study) — 75.00

Dr. Satish Goel
- Causes & Cure of Blood Pressure — 75.00
- Causes & Cure of Diabetes — 60.00
- Causes & Cure of Heart Ailments — 75.00
- Pregnancy & Child Care — 95.00
- Ladie's Slimming Course — 95.00
- Acupuncture Guide — 50.00
- Acupressure Guide — 50.00
- Acupuncture & Acupressure Guide — 95.00
- Walking for Better Health — 95.00
- Nature Cure for Health & Happiness — 95.00
- A Beacon of Hope for the Childless Couples — 60.00
- Sex for All — 75.00

Dr. Kanta Gupta
- Be Your Own Doctor — 60.00
  (a Book about Herbs & Their Use)

Dr. B.R. Kishore
- Vatsyana Kamasutra — 95.00
- The Manual of Sex & Tantra — 95.00

Dr. M.K. Gupta
- Causes, Cure & Prevention of High Blood Cholesterol — 60.00

Acharya Bhagwan Dev
- Yoga for Better Health — 95.00
- Pranayam, Kundalini aur Hathyoga — 60.00

Dr. R.N. Gupta
- Joys of Parenthood — 40.00

M. Kumaria
- How to Keep Fit — 20.00

Dr. Renu Gupta
- Hair Care (Prevention of Dandruff & Baldness) — 75.00
- Skin Care — 75.00
- Complete Beautician Course (Start a Beauty Parlour at Home) — 95.00
- Common Diseases of Women — 95.00

Dr. S.K. Sharma
- Add Inches — 60.00
- Shed Weight Add Life — 60.00
- Alternate Therapies — 95.00
- Miracles of Urine Therapy — 60.00
- Meditation & Dhyan Yoga (for Spiritual Discipline) — 95.00
- A Complete Guide to Homeopathic Remedies — 120.00
- A Complete Guide to Biochemic Remedies — 60.00
- Common Diseases of Urinary System — 95.00
- Allopathic Guide for Common Disorders — 125.00
- E.N.T. & Dental Guide (in Press) — 95.00
- Wonders of Magnetotherapy — 95.00
- Family Homeopathic Guide — 95.00
- Health in Your Hands — 95.00
- Food for Good Health — 95.00
- Juice Therapy — 75.00
- Tips on Sex — 75.00

Dr. Rajiv Sharma
- First Aid (in Press) — 95.00
- Causes, Cure and Prevention of Children's Diseases — 75.00

Dr. Pushpa Khurana
- Be Young and Healthy for 100 Years — 60.00
- The Awesome Challenge of AIDS — 40.00

Acharya Satyanand
- Surya Chikitsa — 95.00

Dr. Nishtha
- Diseases of Respiratory Tract (Nose, Throat, Chest & Lungs) — 95.00
- Backache (Spondylitis, Cervical Arthritis, Rheumatism) — 95.00
- Ladies Health Guide (With Make-up Guide) — 95.00

L.R. Chowdhary
- Rajuvenate with Kundalini Mantra Yoga — 95.00

Manoj Kumar
- Diamond Body Building Course — 95.00

Koulacharya Jagdish Sharma
- Body Language — 125.00

G.C. Goyal
- Vitamins for Natural Healing — 95.00

Dr. Vishnu Jain
- Heart to Heart (with Heart Specialist) — 95.00

Asha Pran
- Beauty Guide (With Make-up Guide) — 75.00

Acharya Vipul Rao
- Ayurvedic Treatment for Common Diseases — 95.00
- Herbal Treatment for Common Diseases — 95.00

Dr. Sajiv Adlakha
- Stuttering & Your Child (Question-Answer) — 60.00

Books can be requisitioned by V.P.P. Postage charges will be Rs. 20/- per book.
For orders of three books the postage will be free.

◉ DIAMOND POCKET BOOKS

X-30, Okhla Industrial Area, Phase-II, New Delhi-110020, Phone : 011-41611861, Fax : 011-41611866
E-mail : sales@dpb.in, Website : www.dpb.in

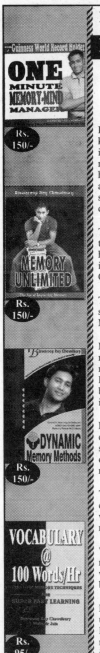
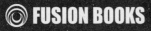

Diamond Books Presents

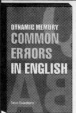

Dynamic Memory Common Errors in English
Tarun Chakarbory
English is a widely used language in our business & professional environment and further in corporate world it is a must. It may be very closely observed that for most of the times, the English used by people is not correct, yet it is spoken and written out of ignorence in the same way. Such show is rated as very bad by learned people.This book by Tarun Chakraborty is a result of his great efforts where he has identified such common errors and presented their correct use. **Rs. 110.00**

Dynamic Memory Perfect Spoken in English
Tarun Chakarbory
English speaking is generally latest as a impressive tool among all class of people. But for most of the times the spoken English is not correct rather it is full of errors. At a glance, such incorrect spoken English is marked behind fluency but it is categoried as a poor show by learned people. This valuable book of Tarun Chakarborty is a meaning full effort to catch the attention of people to correct themselves. The book provides a lot of material to meet the objective. **Rs. 110.00**

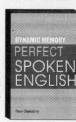

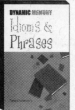

Dynamic Memory Idioms & Phrases
Tarun Chakarbory
This book 'Dynamic Memory Idioms & Phrases' is well written by Sri Tarun Chakraborty to offer a huge collection of idioms, with this idiomatic origin and further their meaning. The idioms are arranged in alphabatic order which is of great help to book user 'the help is further supplemented by content index given at the begin of the book. The book is certainly very valuable for student & English lovers. **Rs. 95.00**

Dynamic Memory Group Discussions
Tarun Chakarbory
Group discussion is a very effective tool to select propes manpower for any good jobs. A candidate has to project his skills of expression to the board, at the same times has to slow that he is good to work in a team, while he is a brilliant leader like person as well. It is a tought experience to overcome group discussion if one is not practical & orient for such game. This book by Tarun Chakarborty steps to predse up this gap and tends to remove the obvious hitch in the candidates. Rs. : 95.00

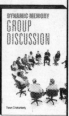

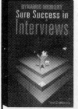

Dynamic Memory Sure Success in Interview
Tarun Chakarbory
When you are invited to an interview it means that the hiring manager believes you may be a good match for the job opening, she or he want to know for sure. This book is a ready reckoner for those who want to present themselves in a powerful & prossive way.
Rs. : 95.00

Dynamic Memory Synoniums & Antonimous Dictionary
Tarun Chakarbory
Communication is effective when we have a firm grip on vocabulary. Anyone should make the reader's job easier by communicating whatever he or she wants to communicate.
Not only does reading allow you to build up your vocabulary, but it also allows you to become more informed, learning things about the world around you. **Rs. : 95.00**

Books can be requisitioned by V.P.P. Postage charges will be Rs. 20/- per book.
For orders of three books the postage will be free.

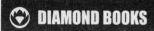

DIAMOND BOOKS   X-30, Okhla Industrial Area, Phase-II, New Delhi-110020,
Phone : 41611861 Fax : 41611866
E-mail : sales@dpb.in Website : www.dpb.in

Best of Indian Classics

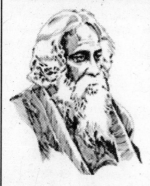

Rabindranath inherited great mind from his father, Maharshi Devendranath Thakur, a religious reformer who expounded Brahmo Samaj (the Society of Lord Brahma).

Rabindranath returned from England without completing studies and started writing poems very early. He captured the rhythm of life from the melody of rain drops, which he composed, developed and researched later. In 1890 his first collection of poems was published, as 'Manasi', which, today critics believe, contained symptoms of his intellectual maturity.

All his life he studied at home, and stopped going to school after seventh standard when he saw class-teachers mercilessly beating students for simple follies. He was naturally learnt. He studied Hindu Scriptures, sciences, and world literatures avidly all his life, but did not take standard university examinations. Despite that, he was the examiner of Calcutta University Bengali Literature answer-scripts, honoured with many honorary doctorates and D Litts., followed by scholars world over in literature and musicology.

He won India's first Nobel Prize in 1913 for 'Gitanjali, Song Offerings', and with the prize money created 'Santiniketan' in Birbhum district of today's West Bengal. Santiniketan translated his vision of education, humanity, rural economy, civil society and research, to disseminate the concept of Visva Bharati, which later became a Central University.

He wrote in all 2,500 lyrics, composed into mellifluous songs which by his nephew Dinendranath Tagore and his first-line disciples, which created a new and universally popular genre in Indian musicology, known as 'Rabindrasangeet'.

Rabindranath Tagore

- Gitanjali
- Gora
- Yogayog
- Aankh Ki Kirkari
- Inside Outside
- Boat Accident
- Choker Bali
- Bau Thakuranir Haat

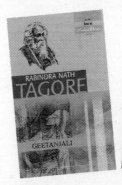
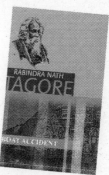

Diamond Books

X-30, Okhla Industrial Area, Phase-II, New Delhi-110020
Ph.: 41611861, Fax: 41611866, E-mail: sales@dpb.in, Website: www.dpb.in

COMPUTER BOOKS

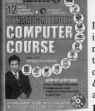

DYNAMIC MEMORY COMPUTER COURSE
Biswaroop Roy Chowdhury

In today's cyber world, not knowing about computer is nothing less than illiteracy. Knowing about computer and its uses is no more a luxury but a necessity. This book has been brought out keeping this necessity in mind. In this book the fantastic story of the computer from its inception to its vital state on covered. Every nuance from hardware to software, interest to networking & from MS-Office to Window XP/Vista, a reader will get all he wants to know about computers.Computer will be as clear as your drinking water.

 Rs. 250.00

Dynamic Memory Windows Vista & Office 2007
Devender Singh Minhas

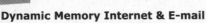

The technology of Windows and internet to computer system has created an open run way for new introductions. In this field as well, every new version overrides old version and comes forward with yet more power & features. *Window Vista* is one such latest version & this book updates its readers, with the novality. Devender Minhas has once again done his wonderful job.

Rs. 200.00

Dynamic Memory Windows 98/XP & Internet
Devender Singh Minhas

In the hi-tech world, not knowing about the computer is nothing less than illiteracy. Computer has become an intergral part of our life. Computer touches our every aspect of life making it easier and comfortable. So, knowing about computer and its uses are no more a knowledge but a necessity. This book has been brought forth keeping this necessity in mind. **Rs. 110.00**

Dynamic Memory Internet & E-mail
Davinder Singh Minhas

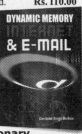

In today's educated world, not knowing about Internet is nothing less than illiteracy. This book will be a handy tool to become an expert on Internet. Every step from the equipments you need to have an Internet to the method of approaching an Internet Service provider. From E-mail to Internet safety and from Web browser to e-commerce, a reader will get all in this book. **Rs. 110.00**

Dynamic Memory Internet Dictionary
Tarun Chakarborty

This Internet Dictionary contains almost all the necessary Internet Terminology. Surely, it will benefit all those who are NET savvy and willing to know more about the endless world of WorldWide Web (WWW). **Rs. 110.00**

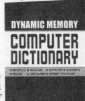

Dynamic Memory Computer Dictionary
Tarun Chakarborty

This dictionary is an essential guide to modern computer terminology and jargon and contains hundreds of straightforward definitions, example sentences and usage tips. The terms are illustrated wherever possible for the convenience of the readers. **Rs. 110.00**

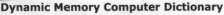

Books can be requisitioned by V.P.P. Postage charges will be Rs. 20/- per book.
For orders of three books the postage will be free.

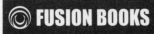

FUSION BOOKS　　X-30, Okhla Industrial Area, Phase-II, New Delhi-110020,
Phone : 41611861 Fax : 41611866
E-mail : sales@dpb.in Website : www.dpb.in